The

Weight Loss Cookbook

By Donald L. Turpin

**A Complete Weight Loss System
With
Accompanying Cookbook
And
Color-Coded Food Selections**

ISBN 978-0-6151-9613-8

Library of Congress Control Number: 2008904397

Dedication

This book is dedicated to **Betty**, my most avid supporter, fan, best lifelong friend, and loving wife.

Acknowledgements

I want to thank the many people who have assisted me over the past two decades by trying the recipes and providing me with suggestions and detailed feedback on the results of the integrated weight loss program. I further appreciate the many recipes that have been submitted to me for analysis and consideration. Many of those have been modified to comply with my weight loss principles and included in this cookbook.

About the Author

Donald, along with his wife Betty, is the previous owner and operator of a highly successful restaurant. He has successfully completed the Department of Health course in proper food handling and storage. Donald earned his Bachelor of Science degree plus his Master's degree in Industrial Technology from Eastern Kentucky University. He then completed an advanced program, above the Master's Degree, at the University of Kentucky. He served as a Commissioned Officer in the United States Army, including the command of food service operations for a large military installation. He also has a great deal of experience as the administrator of food service support services for two large Florida public school districts. He has utilized his experiences and a non-scientific approach to study the realistic effects of foods on weight loss for almost twenty years as of the printing of this edition. His years' of experience in the selection, storage, preparation, and distribution of foods have significantly contributed to the writing of this cookbook. Donald is pleased to share his findings and conclusions with you in the form of this second and expanded edition.

Please keep in mind that while we have studied the results of research on weight loss for almost two decades, have applied common sense and logic to those results, know how to cook foods that promote weight loss, and have documented proof of the positive results of our weight loss recipes and program, the author, no contributor, or member of the Weight Loss Cookbook staff is a doctor or a nutritionist. Therefore, medical issues will not be addressed in this cookbook. Due to the many possible variations of individual health problems, we recommend that you consult your doctor or health care professional prior to implementing **any** exercise routine, weight loss program, or changing your diet; especially if one has been prescribed for you. Please keep in mind that no two people are alike, therefore, the results of this or any other program will vary to some degree from one individual to another.

Contents

Introduction

Losing weight is really a very simple and uncomplicated process. There are only three basic rules which you must follow:

Rule Number One: *You must minimize your consumption of foods that are void of color or that grow below ground.*

Rule Number Two: *You must "refine" less "fuel" than your body uses.*

Rule Number Three: *You must avoid what I call the "Deprivation Syndrome" by eating a minimum of three proper meals per day and by selecting one day per week as a "Free Day" to eat anything that you want.*

These three rules served as guides during the approximately twenty years of research and development for this cookbook. If you will use the specified ingredients, prepare the dishes as instructed and eat only the foods listed in this cookbook, you should lose as much weight as you want like many others have done.

All too often, diet "gurus" will explain, in detail, their theories but leave you with the question, **"But what do I eat?"** I have chosen to take the opposite approach by providing you with dozens of delicious weight loss recipes, without the technical jargon, along with an extensive list of permitted and color-coded foods from which you may choose. When I learned about the culprits that were making me fat, I researched recipes in hundreds of cookbooks, but rarely found a single one that was not loaded with an excessive amount of fat-producing elements. Therefore, I began the time-consuming process of developing and testing my own recipes that excluded the use of most such elements. Although some of the recipes in this cookbook do contain small amounts of carbohydrates, the amounts are insignificant, and therefore non-fattening, when considered in relation to the sum of all the ingredients in the recipe. Also, some carbohydrates become non-fattening when combined with certain other ingredients. This complex combining factor has also been incorporated into the recipes through a color-coding system for your convenience.

In summary my proven weight loss theories have been integrated into the recipes in this cookbook; therefore, there is no need for you to be concerned about the technical aspects of losing weight. Just follow the recipes and enjoy the delicious comfort foods while you lose to your goal weight.

What People are Saying!

The many people who have tried it during the past decade can best explain the Weight Loss Cookbook's success. The following are only a few of the many documented statements that we have received down through the years:

"THANK YOU VERY MUCH FOR THE DELICIOUS RECIPES"

"I especially love the lasagna and the breakfast casserole. After I had the kids I ballooned up to 198 pounds at my heaviest. I had tried dieting before... I had really begun to think that my body was just too old or stubborn or whatever. I always gave up... Everyone who sees me mentions my weight loss. It is obvious in the way I look, the way I feel, and the way my clothes feel. I am down to 157... It's a miracle!!!!! Thank you for your help." T. Roberts

"...HIS CHOLESTEROL LEVEL DROPPED..."

"My husband has never had a cholesterol problem. His count has always been around 183 – 189. I was interested to see what his cholesterol level would be after we had eaten eggs, bacon, cheese, etc., on a regular basis. I am pleased to report that his cholesterol level dropped to 149. We were both astonished, because we have been eating what "normally" would be considered high cholesterol foods." Linda

"MY CRAVINGS HAVE ALL GONE, THANKS TO THE FREE DAY!"

"Just wanted to let you know that I have lost 3 pounds my first week. I also want to tell you about my "Free Day." First of all, I think that it is great! I honestly believe that this could very well be the main reason that I could not stick to a weight loss program before now. There is no way that I can tell you how horrible I felt after eating all that stuff that I thought I wanted. My cravings have all gone, thanks to the "Free Day!" D. Iness

"I HAD LOST OVER 45 POUNDS"

"I have been on many diets in my life, and none have worked for me (except this one). In fact, I don't consider this a diet but a way of life that is easy to live with because I am never hungry and I feel great. I had to go to the doctor this month for my annual checkup. Guess what? I had lost over 45 pounds. He couldn't believe it. I am so pleased…not only do I look better, but I feel so much better." Carman S.

"I AM NEVER HUNGRY"

"I am never hungry on your diet and this is why I believe that everyone can stick with your plan. I have lost 22 pounds in 4 months." Richard B.

"THANK YOU FOR GIVING US BACK OUR LIVES"

"I had to take this opportunity to thank you for your wonderful food program. Bill, Eric and I are all doing great. Eric has gone from 218 pounds in June to 178 pounds (his goal weight) on October 1st. Bill has gone from 321 pounds to 295 pounds since June and his cholesterol has gone from 245 to 134 since the end of July. His doctor was absolutely amazed. Thank you again for giving us back our lives." Bill, Barbara and Eric

"MY TRUE REWARD IS HAVING A HEALTHY BODY, MIND AND SPIRIT"

"Week 20, I lost my first 32 pounds and I got my reward, but the best reward is that I am 32 pounds closer to my ultimate goal. My true reward is having a healthy body, mind and spirit! I also want to tell you about my "free day." First of all, I think that it is great! I honestly believe that this could very well be the main reason that I could not stick to a weight loss program before now. There is no way that I can tell you how horrible I felt after eating all that stuff that I thought I wanted. My cravings have all gone, thanks to the "free day!" Debra I

"I HAVE KEPT IT OFF"

"I reached, and still am at, my goal weight by losing 48 pounds within 6 months after beginning the program – that was 9 years ago and I have kept it off. There is just no excuse for you to be fat anymore." Don

"I LOST ALMOST 50 POUNDS BY FOLLOWING ONLY YOUR RULE NO. 1"

"I really started thinking about you telling me that if I eat more than I needed, the extra had to go somewhere. It didn't take me long to figure out that this was the reason that I was just plain fat. I lost almost 50 pounds by following only your Rule No. "1" and by using the recipes in your cookbook." Chet

"Food" for Thought

By Donald L. Turpin

If you are overweight and searching for a way to lose weight, like two-thirds of the people in this country, there are literally millions of diet pills, plans, equipment, meetings, calorie counters, explanations, and schemes designed to take your money from you. To confirm this point, I recently checked the Internet for current selections of possible programs and gimmicks claiming that they have the secrets of weight loss to share with you, for a price of course. Using a major search engine, I searched for the subject of "diet." I was presented with more than 315,000,000 (**three hundred and fifteen million**) possibilities. Using the same search engine, I then searched the web for the term, "weight loss." I was given more than 178,000,000 (**one hundred and seventy eight million**) possibilities. Realizing that you probably won't live long enough to check out all those millions upon millions of possibilities, I suppose another approach would be for you to try the programs that appear to be the most advertised. I know because several years ago I spent a lot of time, as well as a lot of money, on some of those well-known programs in my efforts to lose weight. I would lose a couple of pounds only to gain back three. If you have done the same, you probably understand the frustration that I experienced. I finally gave up on all those "yo-yo" programs and after almost twenty years of my own research on the subject, I have developed a detailed low-carbohydrate weight loss program of my own that has been very effective for me as well as a lot of other people.

The many delicious recipes in this cookbook are based on the results of almost two decades of research which indicates that the human body is a complex "refinery" that refines (metabolizes) raw materials (food) into body fuel (glucose). The body then uses (burns) this fuel, or, the body's fuel system value operator (insulin) permits it to be stored in fat cells (in the form of glycogen.) We have identified those <u>raw materials</u>, the methods of <u>preparation</u>, and the <u>combinations</u> thereof which refine into the most and into the least amount of fuel. What follows is very simple; **this cookbook contains recipes and a list of foods with ingredients that refine into the least amount of fuel, and, which maximizes your body's need to convert your stored fuel into usable fuel thereby causing you to lose weight and keep it off naturally.**

I lost 58 pounds, and have kept it off for many years, by following the three basic and simple rules of my weight loss program that has been incorporated into the recipes of this cookbook. I highly recommend that you read the **What People Are Saying** part of this cookbook to learn how my easy approach has impacted the lives of others.   You too can lose weight simply by preparing and eating the **delicious comfort foods** in this cookbook.

If my three basic rules in the **Introduction** section of this cookbook sound interesting to you, and seem to be ones that you can live with, then read on because I shall briefly explain each of them below:

My first rule requires you to minimize your consumption of foods that are void of color or that grow below ground. I realize that there are many of you out there who are inquisitive individuals, like my wife Betty, and really want an answer to the question, "why?" Therefore, let me now summarize, in non-technical terms, how simple the basis for this rule really is.   One day while I was researching the results of tests that determine, on a scale from 0 to 100, the amount of glucose (body fuel) that the body metabolizes (refines) from various foods and recipe ingredients, my wife Betty observed over my shoulder for a while and then her natural curiosity overtook her. She asked, "What are you doing?" I very proudly showed her some of the results of my efforts over the past few years and explained that I was studying the Glycemic Index (G.I.) in order to determine which foods and ingredients to include in my recipes in order to lose weight. Boy, did she bring this complex matter down to earth by reducing it to its lowest form of understanding. She made a statement that summarizes all my findings in the very best possible way and in the fewest words. She said, "Do you realize that every one of those that you have identified as being fattening are either white or grow below ground?" I immediately realized that she was, for the most part, absolutely correct.   Now talking about putting some technical "stuff" in simple and easy-to-understand terms, that is how it is done! I could have kept this little secret to myself, and explained my concept in the usual complex terms like most researchers, but I decided to share it with you in the form of this cookbook. Think about it for a minute. What foods are white? Flour, corn, sugar, and rice cakes, for example you say. You need to know that all of these are at the top of the list of fattening foods and have therefore been excluded from my recipes.

Let us now consider the question, "What grows below ground?" Potatoes, beets, and carrots for example you say? Oh yea, I know what you're thinking, carrots aren't fattening! Wrong, they too are right at the top of the list along with cake and potatoes when it comes to "refining" into an excessive amount of "body fuel." I'm sure that by now you are beginning to understand why and how I so carefully chose and combined the ingredients for my recipes in this cookbook.

This first rule is based on the simple theory that you must eat low-carbohydrate foods in order to lose weight. **Even if you are on another low-carbohydrate weight loss or diabetic program, I believe that you will find this cookbook to be an outstanding compliment to your success.** I am frequently asked if my weight loss concepts are the same as those of The Atkins Diet. Actually they are similar but certainly not the same. I have answered that question in more detail, plus many others, in the *Frequently Asked Questions* section of this cookbook.

Now let us briefly examine my second rule which pertains to **portion control** for weight loss. Simply put, if you eat more than is required to refine the fuel needed for your daily activities, the excess will be stored in your fat cells; after all, it can't overflow like fuel from the tank of your vehicle. There would be no overweight people if our human "tank" capacities were fixed rather than flexible, but unfortunately, that is not the case. The challenge is to balance your food consumption with your fuel needs, but at the same time, avoid ever being hungry. A simple serving size guide has been included in the *Helpful Guides* section of this cookbook. If you want to lose weight and keep it off, you must become aware of serving sizes and practice portion control. My brother lost over 50 pounds by following this one simple rule.

My third rule is to avoid, what I call, the **"Deprivation Syndrome."** In my opinion this is a natural psychological double-edged sword that can seriously interfere with your weight loss efforts. Therefore, you must avoid this condition by selecting one day per week as a **"Free Day"** to eat anything that you want; that's right, **anything that you want!**

If you are ever going to lose weight and keep it off, you must understand the significance of, and avoid, the Deprivation Syndrome. First of all, if your body senses that you are not getting enough food, it will go into a mode of making as much body fuel out of what you do eat as it can. Of the past few million years of food intake by humans, only the last few have provided us with such a huge quantity, variety and combination of foods. Human bodies haven't had enough time to adjust to such luxury. Therefore, when you cut back too drastically on food, your body will prepare for a famine, the same as it would have done a thousand years ago, by going into the Deprivation Syndrome. Simple, but makes a lot of sense, don't you agree? Now, for the first tip to help you avoid the deprivation syndrome; **do not skip meals!** Too often people get "stuck" at a weight and can't seem to lose any more. What do they do? They start skipping meals based on the belief that they have been eating too much of the wrong food. This is perhaps one of the worse mistakes that one can make when trying to lose weight. The body thinks, "Well, here we go again, must be a bad year for nuts and berries, so I need to reduce energy and stock up by storing all the body fuel that I can make into the ole fat cells." Guess what happens next. You are right; you do not lose any more weight. As a matter of fact, you might even gain a pound or two even though you are eating less of the proper foods. Then what happens? You become frustrated, give up, abandon the program, and become fatter and fatter. This is the primary reason that people weigh more shortly after giving up on a diet than they did before going on the diet. As you probably know, most fat people have tried a diet, at some time or another, which did not work for them. When you reach a plateau where you are not losing weight, just hang in there and **don't deviate from my three basic rules**. When your body learns that it really is not going to starve to death, it will revert back to a normal status and you will start losing weight again.

Secondly, I believe that most people don't stay on a chosen weight loss program because they reach a point where they feel overwhelmingly "deprived" of the so-called "fattening" and "good-tasting" foods. At such times, it is easy to develop the attitude, "What the heck, life is short and I am going to enjoy it even if it does mean being fat." You can avoid such an attitude and easily continue your weight loss if you will select one day of each week to eat anything that you want. I call this my *"Free Day"* concept, which by the way, is one of the most important long-term parts of my weight loss program. You are probably thinking to yourself, "Yea right, come on now!" Now hear me out on this one because you will be glad that you did. If you divide all the food that you eat in one week by seven days, you will learn that one day represents only about 14 percent of the total for that week. Now here is my reasoning behind this idea; if you cut out 86 percent of the fattening foods that you now eat, your body will not think that it is starving to death and develop the Deprivation Syndrome. There are actually three very good reasons for the Free Day: (1) you will enjoy so-called fattening foods, (2) you will lose weight, and (3) you will not be likely to abandon the program. Do not think that you can skip the Free Day and still lose weight, or even stay on any program, for very long. Enjoy your Free Day, but be forewarned, you will not feel very well, physically that is, after you eat all that food and in the combinations that you thought you wanted. However, this too is good because it will result in you realizing how bad your food choices probably have been in the past and still are at the present time.

For years, my slim, trim and thankful friends kept telling me that I should write a cookbook and integrate my simple weight loss concepts into the recipes. Well, here it is. If you use these recipes, lose a lot of weight and find yourself being chased for your body, don't blame me. Betty and our friends talked me into it. Meanwhile, I plan to add many more good weight loss recipes for comfort foods to this cookbook during the years to come. Therefore, your feedback in the form of comments, questions, success stories, and any suggested recipes are welcome. Feel free to email them to me at www.donaldturpin@hotmail.com.

Frequently Asked Questions (FAQ)

During the past several years, I have been asked several questions about the recipes in this cookbook; however an overwhelming majority of the questions have been about my weight loss program that inspired it. I would like to use this means of sharing several of the most frequently asked questions, and my answers to those questions with you, as follows:

QUESTION: *The weight loss concepts behind your recipes and the concepts of "The Atkins Diet" appear to be similar. Are they the same?*

ANSWER: First of all, let me say that I am not trying to sell you a diet plan. Secondly, I don't know how long that Dr. Atkins has been developing his program, but I have been working on mine for almost 20 years as of the date of this edition. I have read his book and apparently the concepts are similar, but they certainly are not the same. Although both are based on the need to restrict such foods as sugar, breads, pasta, cereal, starchy vegetables, etc, my cookbook concentrates on **what** and **when** you can eat to lose weight rather than on technical subjects. In my opinion, my program is much simpler and easier to follow without giving up on your efforts. Furthermore, I have concentrated on **comfort foods that you can enjoy**. I seriously doubt if you will even know that you are on a diet when you eat dishes prepared by my proven recipes.

QUESTION: *Can you provide me with some guidelines on the amount of bread that I may have with a meal? Also, is there a limit?*

ANSWER: Yes, there is a limit. Bread is white isn't it? I believe that I need to expand a little on this subject. It has been reported that 9 out of every 10 people eat flour in some form with every meal. If you will just look around, you probably can easily identify the 9 people. Flour, in any form, is very fattening and must be avoided, except on your Free Day, if you ever hope to lose a significant amount of weight. This includes crackers, pretzels, bagels, breaded foods, cake, cookies, donuts, pancakes, pie crust, etc. However, there is a bread that you can use as you like. It can be found in most health food stores and major chain food stores. The name of the bread is *Ezekiel 4:9*, the ingredients of which are derived from the same chapter and verse in *The Bible*. It is baked by the *Food for Life* bakery. *Ezekiel 4:9* is made from live sprouted grains and is 100% flourless and sugar free. As odd as it may seem, the combination of grains in the bread creates a protein very similar to that of meat, eggs, milk and cheese. Therefore, I treat it as a protein (color coded red), rather than a carbohydrate, in my weight loss system and cookbook.

QUESTION: *You stated that if it is white or if it grows below ground, do not combine it with any animal or fish product. Why is that?*

ANSWER: The facts that support this concept are really very simple. You see, the body requires the secretion of an acid type enzyme to refine (metabolize) the animal product and the secretion of an alkaline type enzyme to refine the other foods. These two enzymes are not that much unlike acid and vinegar. When mixed together, the two tend to neutralize each other and therefore neither is effective in accomplishing its intended purpose. Thus the meat rots and the other foods ferment and cause gas. I could carry this on to the point of being gross, but I will leave that to your imagination. I will, however, add that not much "refining" can take place under such conditions. Therefore the digestive process can take twice as long as normal. Meanwhile, you have rotten food working its way through your colon. I happen to believe that colon cancer, plus other health problems, such as "heartburn," can result from such poor eating habits.

QUESTION: *What do you suggest that I eat as a snack?*

ANSWER: Nothing! The refining process can be drastically upset by a snack eaten between meals. Just think through this with me for a moment. After you eat a meal, the body will analyze the food to determine if an acid type enzyme or an alkaline type enzyme will be required to break the food down and perform the refining process. Once the determination is made, the correct enzyme is secreted and the refining process begins. Now lets consider what happens if you eat a snack during this refining process. I believe that the body should be able to yell out, "What are you doing? About the time I get going on this refining business, you dump some other food product down here for me to analyze, causing me to have to start the process all over again." It has been reported that, on the average, it takes the body approximately three hours to refine a meal and send it on its way in the form of energy. I suggest that you leave your digestive system alone during that three hours and let it do its job as intended by not messing things up with a snack.

QUESTION: *I have always been told that I must cut down on fat and burn calories in order to lose weight. What is your response to that advice?*

ANSWER: I personally am not concerned about "fat" or "calories" like most researchers. My conclusions are based on **my** years of research into the matters of how the body metabolizes so-called fat and the calorie theory that was established back in 1935. I have no desire to argue the point but you must realize that "we have come a long way baby" since then. In my opinion, the calorie theory is as much out of date as the horse and buggy. I happen to believe that the body doesn't "burn" anything. Instead, it simply **refines** raw products, known as food, into body fuel, which is glucose. It then stores the excess glucose, which we do not use, in the form of glycogen in our fat cells. But of course, it is all right if you disagree with me on these matters because if you use my recipes to prepare your meals, you should still lose weight.

QUESTION: *Is it OK to eat potatoes as long as they are baked?*

ANSWER: If you are going to lose weight, you must not eat potatoes, except on your Free Day, regardless of how they are prepared. Potatoes rank near the top of the list of "fuel-making" foods. Our objective is to cause your body to "refine" less "fuel" and then to use that which is now stored in your fat cells. Hopes this helps.

QUESTION: *One of my coworkers skips lunch occasionally and eats some light microwave popcorn instead. Is this a good way to lose some weight?*

ANSWER: Absolutely not! Popcorn is right up at the top of the list when it comes to fattening foods, especially when it is eaten by itself. After all, it is white isn't it? Now let me ask you, are the people who eat popcorn for lunch fat? Now another question for you, what do farmers feed cattle to fatten them up for market? Corn of course; I rest my case.

QUESTION: *I have heard that it is important to drink a considerable amount of water in order to lose weight. Is this true?*

ANSWER: Yes, it is true. Researchers tell us that you should drink a minimum of 6 glasses of water per day in order to lose much weight. Water with lemon is recommended. Some research indicates that a teaspoon of lemon juice with a meal can reduce the fattening effects of that meal by as much as thirty percent. Try to drink as little as possible with meals in order to avoid interfering with the metabolizing process.

QUESTION: *Should I eat fruit while I am trying to lose weight?*

ANSWER: Yes, you should eat fruit because it is good for you. However, the timing for eating fruit is extremely important. First of all, it should never be combined with any other food, even on your Free Day. Here is my recommendation; never eat any fruit within 3 hours after a meal, and never eat a meal within 45 minutes after eating fruit. This is because fruit metabolizes within 45 minutes, and it takes 3 hours to metabolize a regular meal. Fruit is simply not compatible with any other food. As a matter of fact, I recommend that you don't even combine fruits because of their differences. Apply these same rules to fruit juices.

QUESTION: *Is alcohol fattening?*

ANSWER: Yes it is. The adverse effect of alcohol on weight control becomes even more pronounced when it is mixed with a sweetened mix such as a cola. Alcohol is quickly absorbed into the bloodstream, resulting in a rapid increase of insulin, the fat-storing enzyme. Beer (maltose) for example, is 14% more fattening than potatoes and 32% more fattening than refined sugar. However, I am of the opinion that one glass of dry (un-sweet) red wine with a meal is acceptable. It has been reported that the tannin in a glass of red wine will decrease the bad cholesterol (LDL) level.

QUESTION: *Do colas really contain a lot of sugar?*

ANSWER: If you will check the label of a well-known cola, you probably will find that it contains 39 grams of sugar. **That is 9 ¾ teaspoons of sugar per can.** Research also indicates that the other contents of a soft drink can easily interfere with your food refining process by causing a chemical imbalance in your system. I recommend that you drink a diet version of soft drink, but better yet, omit them from your diet altogether and enjoy a cool glass of water with lemon instead.

QUESTION: *How often should I weight myself and how should I keep track of my weight loss progress?*

ANSWER: I recommend that you do not weigh yourself each day, because if you do, you will frequently be disappointed. Instead, consider your weight loss as a long-term project and weigh yourself no more than once every two to three weeks. You will know when you are losing weight because your clothes will start to fall off you. If you use the recipes in this cookbook for your meals, and if you follow my recommendations, you should lose an average of 1 to 3 pounds per week. You didn't put it all on in a short time and you should not take it off in a short time. The objective is to lose fat, not muscle.

QUESTION: *I suffer from heartburn most of the time. Is this possibly the result of bad food combinations?*

ANSWER: I don't know, but it could very well be, especially if you are combining such foods as a steak and potato or eating meat sandwiches for example. In such cases, gas from the fermenting potato or bread pushes the acid needed to metabolize the meat back up from the stomach into your esophagus causing heartburn. Furthermore, gas created from the rotting meat and fermenting carbohydrate can result in bad breath plus a lot of other uncomfortable and embarrassing problems. As always, I recommend that you consult with your doctor if your problem persists because you could have a medical problem rather than a food combination related problem.

QUESTION: *I love your recipes but I work and have to eat out in restaurants a lot. What can I do to stay on your weight loss concept?*

ANSWER: You are not unlike a lot of other people that have fulltime jobs. A recent study indicates that the average American dines in restaurants four times per week. I believe that the best advice that I can give you is to prepare extra food by my recipes and take your lunch, or dinner, to work with you. Most workplaces now have microwaves and refrigerators to accommodate employees. Realizing that you cannot always do that, my next best recommendation is for you to ask for what you want when ordering in a restaurant rather than accepting a fattening dish that is offered to you. In most restaurants, you will first be served bread and butter, a very bad combination and very fattening, especially when consumed on an empty stomach. In most instances, the digesting (refining) of the bread and butter will have already begun before you receive your main meal. When ordering, you will also probably be asked to choose either a baked potato or fries as a side item. So goes the process of choosing between two equally fattening foods. Now, let me give you an example of how to handle a situation like this. First of all, do not eat the bread, period. When you place your order, simply **ask** for a side item such as steamed vegetables or a side salad. You pay for your meal so why shouldn't you have the right to make the decisions about the food to eat that will result in you losing weight?

QUESTION: *If I prepare my meals by your recipes, will I still need to exercise to lose weight?*

ANSWER: You probably will still lose weight, however, exercising is highly recommended to "tone" your body and muscles as you lose weight. Also remember that an idling engine uses very little fuel and unused body fuel is stored in your fat cells. Exercising helps to burn the excess fuel, but more importantly, it helps your body to become efficient in the refining of raw products (food). Research indicates that a schedule of brisk walking for at least 30 minutes each day is perhaps the best exercise routine that one can follow. However, I realize that everyone is subject to various physical restrictions; therefore, I highly recommend that you consult your doctor about an exercise routine that is best for you.

QUESTION: *I use a great deal of honey as a sweetener. Is it fattening like sugar?*

ANSWER: In my opinion, you should avoid all sugar, syrups, honey, and molasses to the extent possible. Also, I recommend that you develop the habit of reading labels on prepared and canned foods for the purpose of determining sugar content. The average consumption of sugar for every man, woman and child in this country is 149 pounds per year – that is over 10 pounds per month for each. Most of this, I might ad, is in the prepared foods that people eat. I also recommend that you use artificial sweeteners sparingly. The body has a tendency to interpret such sweeteners as being sugar, and it therefore produces an excessive amount of insulin which permits too much of the meal to be stored as fat. Try to gradually cut back on your sugar consumption. You will be surprised how little you do need.

Guide for Using the Recipe and Food Choice Color-Codes

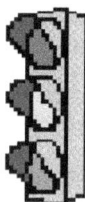

Research indicates that the combination of foods and the ingredients in recipes significantly impact their effects on one's weight. For example, when bread is dipped in olive oil, as is often the case in Italian restaurants, the glycemic factor of the bread is reduced to the extent that its fattening effect is minimized to an acceptable level; as long as the bread is eaten in moderation and in combination with a full meal of other carefully selected foods. Therefore the first major task in this area was to determine, through further research, which recipes could be combined into a meal that will enhance weight loss.

When you consider the large number of different types of foods and the possible combinations of ingredients in recipes, you begin to develop an understanding of the complexity involved in this principle. I realized that I must develop recipes with the proper combinations of ingredients; which I have done for those in this cookbook. I further realized that I must find a way to properly combine the completed dishes in such a way that it could be universally understood. One day while waiting my turn at a stop light, it dawned on me that the colors on stop lights, red, yellow, and green, were in the same location on every stop light throughout the country. My observation resulted in the idea of color-coding recipes by using the colors and locations of those colors on a stoplight. As it became more universally used, I began to realize that this unique system of combining foods could very well be one of the major keys to the success of the weight loss program. Therefore, I have integrated it throughout this cookbook by color-coding all the recipes and list of permitted foods for your convenience.

Now, let me explain how my simple **Stoplight System** of choosing dishes works. As you know, the top color of a traffic light is red, the middle color is yellow, and the bottom color is green. The red and the green do not touch, yet the red and yellow touch; and, the yellow and green touch. Using the above traffic light as a guide, here is how it works:

1. If a recipe or food item of your choice is color-coded **red**, you may combine it with any other which is also coded red; or, you may combine it with any choice color-coded yellow. But you should not combine it with any choice color-coded green because red and green are separated by yellow on the stoplight.

2. If a recipe or food item of your choice is color-coded **yellow**, you may combine it with any other that is also coded yellow.

3. If a recipe or food item of your choice is color-coded **green**, you may combine it with any other which is also coded green; or, you may combine it with any choice color-coded yellow. But you should not combine it with any choice color-coded red because green and red are separated by yellow on the stoplight.

In summary, avoid combining any recipes or food items that are color-coded red with any that are color-coded green. Such combinations will be detrimental to your weight loss efforts. All other combinations are acceptable.

Companion Recipes

Category of Recipe: | Appetizer

Name of Recipe: | Roasted Pecans

Recipe Color Code: | Yellow

Ingredients:

1 – pound pecan halves
½ - pound butter, melted
1 – teaspoon salt

Instructions:

Preheat oven to 250 degrees. Place the pecan halves on a non-greased cookie sheet with sides. Salt pecans to taste and evenly pour the melted butter over the pecans. Bake until evenly browned, about 25 minutes. Must stir pecans every 4 minutes to prevent burning. Can be stored in a tin.
Serves 10 to 12

Category of Recipe: Appetizer

Name of Recipe: Olive Roll-Ups

Recipe Color Code: Red

Ingredients:

3 – boiled ham, medium thickness
2 – tablespoons whipped cream cheese
24 – pimiento-stuffed green olives
24 – cocktail picks

Instructions:

Evenly spread a generous ½ tablespoon cream cheese on each of the 4 slices of boiled ham. Evenly cut each of the 4 slices of ham into strips. Wrap each of the strips around an olive. Cocktail picks may be used to secure the wraps.
Serves 24

Category of Recipe: | Appetizer

Name of Recipe: | Shrimp Cocktail

Recipe Color Code: | Red

Ingredients:

1 – cup coarsely chopped tomato
½ - cup finely chopped onion
¼ - cup chopped cilantro (or snipped parsley)
1 ½ - tablespoons finely chopped canned green chili
    peppers.
2 – tablespoons cooking oil
2 – tablespoons lime juice
1/2 – teaspoon salt
1/4 – teaspoon black pepper
1 – cup shredded lettuce
1 – pound large fresh or frozen shrimp; shelled,
    de-veined, cooked and chilled

Instructions:

Combine first 8 ingredients and mix thoroughly. Cover and chill in refrigerator for a minimum of 2 hours. Place lettuce, evenly divided, in 8 cocktail glasses. Arrange shrimp, also evenly divided, on top of lettuce. Spoon a tablespoon of the tomato mixture over the shrimp in each of the glasses.
Serves 8

Category of Recipe: | Appetizer

Name of Recipe: | Beer Cheese (dip or spread)

Recipe Color Code: | Red

Ingredients:

1 - 16 ounce package of Velveeta cheese
4 - Ounces cottage cheese
3/4 - Cup shredded cheddar cheese
1 - Tablespoon crushed red pepper
2 - Cloves garlic, crushed
1 - Teaspoon dry mustard
1 - Tablespoon hot Hungarian paprika (or mild if choice)
1 - Can flat warm beer

Instructions:

Set Velveeta cheese and opened can of beer out the night before. Place cottage cheese into food processor and process until smooth; transfer to small bowl and set aside. Place Velveeta cheese in food processor and process until smooth. Add the processed cottage cheese, along with all the spices, and process for 1 minute. Add cheddar cheese and a small amount of beer; process for one additional minute. Continue to add beer until the mixture is a desired consistency. Process until cheese is smooth and creamy. Spices may be adjusted to taste.
Serves 8 to 12

Note: This dip, or spread, will be the talk of the party!

Category of Recipe: Appetizer

Name of Recipe: Portabella Mushrooms

Recipe Color Code: Red

Ingredients:

6 - Large Portabella mushrooms
2 - Tablespoons sugar-free salsa or pizza sauce
3 - Plum tomatoes, sliced
6 - Slices baked ham, cut into thin strips or bite size
pieces
3/4 - Cup shredded provolone, cheddar, or mozzarella
cheese
1/4 - Cup olive oil
1/4 - Teaspoon ground black pepper
1/2 - Teaspoon basil
1/2 - Teaspoon thyme
1/2 - Teaspoon salt

Instructions:

Pre-heat oven to 350 degrees. Lightly brush top and
bottom of mushrooms with olive oil. Place mushrooms
on a baking sheet or in a baking dish. Equally divide
salsa or sauce onto mushrooms. Sprinkle with black
pepper, basil, thyme, and salt to taste. Divide tomatoes
and ham into 6 equal parts and place on the mushrooms.
Equally divide cheese onto top of mushrooms. Bake at
350 degrees for 15 minutes.
Serves 6

Category of Recipe: | Appetizer |

Name of Recipe: | Broccamole Dip |

Recipe Color Code: | Yellow |

Ingredients:

4 - Broccoli stems without florets, chopped
1 - Tablespoon lemon juice
1/4 - Teaspoon ground cumin
1/8 - Teaspoon garlic powder
1 - Small tomato, diced
1 - 4 ounce can green chilies, chopped

Instructions:

Over high heat, bring pot of water to boil. Add broccoli and cook until tender (6 to 7 minutes) and drain. In food processor, combine broccoli, lemon juice, cumin, and garlic powder. Process until smooth. Transfer to bowl, stir in tomato and chilies. Chill until ready to serve. Serves 6 to 8

Category of Recipe: | Appetizer

Name of Recipe: | Cheese Ball

Recipe Color Code: | Red

Ingredients:

1 - 8 ounce cream cheese
1 - Clove garlic, crushed
1 - Teaspoon basil
1 - Teaspoon caraway seed
1 - Teaspoon chives
1 - Teaspoon dill weed
1/4 - Teaspoon lemon pepper

Instructions:

Mix all ingredients, except lemon pepper, and make into balls. Sprinkle lemon pepper over cheese balls.
Serves 6

Category of Recipe: Appetizer

Name of Recipe: Crab Dip

Recipe Color Code: Red

Ingredients:

1 - 8 ounce package Philadelphia Brand cream cheese,
    room temperature
1/4 - Cup canola oil mayonnaise
1 - 6 ounce can white chunk crab meat, drained
3 - Tablespoons capers, drained

Instructions:

Place cream cheese, mayonnaise, and caper in blender.
Blend until capers are chopped. Add crab meat and stir
with spatula.
Serves 4 to 6

Category of Recipe: | Appetizer

Name of Recipe: | Smoked Salmon Dip

Recipe Color Code: | Red

Ingredients:

1 - 14.75 Oz. can salmon
5 – heaping Tablespoons mayonnaise
3 – teaspoons lemon juice
1 ¼ - teaspoons liquid smoke
1 – teaspoon minced garlic
1 – teaspoon prepared horse radish
1 – teaspoon Dijon mustard

Instructions:

Drain salmon. In a large mixing bowl, and using a heavy wire whisk, mash and mix all the ingredients together to a smooth consistency. Serve as a dip or on crackers of choice.
Serves 8 to 10

Category of Recipe: | Beef

Name of Recipe: | Burgers with Butter Sauce

Recipe Color Code: | Red

Ingredients:

2 - Pounds ground chuck
1 - Medium onion, chopped
1/4 - Cup green onions, chopped
2 - Large eggs
3 - Teaspoons Worcestershire sauce
1 - Tablespoon fresh parsley, chopped
1 - Teaspoon salt
1/2 - Teaspoon ground black pepper
For the sauce:
    3/4 - Cup butter
    2 - Tablespoon Worcestershire sauce
    1 - Cup meat juices (may substitute beef broth)
    1 - Teaspoon fresh parsley, chopped

Instructions:

Preheat broiler. Combine all ingredients, mix well and form into 6 burger patties. Broil in a broiler pan until patties are cooked to desired doneness. Reserve the cooking juices for preparing the accompanying sauce. Prepare the sauce by cooking the butter over medium heat until golden brown. Stir in the Worcestershire sauce and meat juices and cook for 1 minute. Add the parsley and keep the sauce warm until serving. Place the cooked burgers on serving plates. Drizzle each burger with the sauce and serve.
Serves 6

Category of Recipe: Beef

Name of Recipe: Baked Veal Chops

Recipe Color Code: Red

Ingredients:

4 - Veal chops, about 14 ounces each
2 - Medium tomatoes, peeled and chopped
1 - Tablespoon parsley, finely chopped
1 - Garlic clove, minced
1/2 - Cup white wine
1/4 - Cup green bell pepper, finely chopped
1/4 - Cup onion, finely chopped
1 - Teaspoon dried thyme
1 - Teaspoon dried oregano
Salt to taste
Pepper to taste

Instructions:

Preheat broiler. Salt and pepper the chops to taste.
Broil under high heat on both sides until brown. In a pan,
sauté tomatoes, wine, green pepper, onion, garlic,
parsley, thyme and oregano and simmer for 5 minutes.
Preheat oven to 350 degrees. Spray a baking dish with
non-stick spray. Place the chops in the baking dish and
cover them with the tomato mixture. Bake until the
chops are cooked through.
Serves 4

Category of Recipe: Beef

Name of Recipe: Steak with Onions and Herbs

Recipe Color Code: Red

Ingredients:

1 - Cup tomato juice
1 - Tablespoon olive oil
1/2 - Teaspoon dried basil, crushed
1/2 - Teaspoon dried oregano, crushed
1/4 - Teaspoon ground black pepper
1 - Clove garlic, minced
1 - Pound top round steak, cut 1 inch thick
2 - Large onions, thinly sliced and separated into rings

Instructions:

For marinade, combine tomato juice, oil, basil, oregano, pepper, and garlic; set aside. Trim fat from steak and cut steak into four equal portions. Place meat in a plastic bag set in a deep bowl. Pour marinade over steak. Seal bag; turn to coat steak well. Marinate overnight in the refrigerator. Then, drain steak, reserving marinade. Place onions on an 18 inch square of heavy aluminum foil. Turn edges of foil up slightly. Drizzle 1/2 cup of the reserved marinade over onions. Fold foil tightly to seal. Grill onion packet and steak on an uncovered grill directly over medium coals for 10 minutes. Turn onion packet and steak; brush steak with marinade. Grill steak to desired doneness. Grill onions 8 minutes more or until tender. Unwrap onions and place on a serving plate. Arrange meat atop onion. Spoon any remaining sauce from onions over the meat.
Serves 4

Category of Recipe: | Beef

Name of Recipe: | Double Cheese Burger

Recipe Color Code: | Red

Ingredients:

1 - Pound ground beef
1 - Tablespoon Worcestershire sauce
2 - Scallions, chopped
1 - Tablespoon fresh parsley, chopped
1/2 - Teaspoon salt
1/4 - Teaspoon ground black pepper
8 - Ounces cheddar cheese block, divided
1/2 - Cup heavy cream
1/2 - Teaspoon dry mustard
1/4 - Teaspoon paprika
1 - Egg yolk

Instructions:

In a bowl, combine the first 6 ingredients. Cut half of the cheese block into 1/2 inch thick slices. Form beef mixture into 8 patties. Place 1 slice of cheese in the center of 1 beef patty. Top with another beef patty; pinch sides together to seal in the cheese. Press together sides of burgers to round the edges. Repeat with remaining patties and cheese. In skillet, over medium-high heat, cook burgers until desired doneness is reached (about 4/12 minutes per side for rare). Transfer burgers to serving platter; keep warm. Shred remaining cheese. In a pot, combine cheese, cream, mustard, paprika and 1/4 cup water. Cook, stirring, over medium-low heat until cheese melts. In a bowl, gradually whisk 2 tablespoons hot cheese mixture into egg yolk. Gradually whisk yolk-cheese mixture into cheese mixture; cook until cheese sauce thickens. Serve sauce with burgers.
Serves 4

Category of Recipe:	Beef
Name of Recipe:	Easy Crock Pot Roast Beef
Recipe Color Code:	Red

Ingredients:

2 1/2 - Pounds chuck or rump beef roast
2 - Pouches dried onion soup mix
1 - 14 1/2 ounce can beef broth
1 1/2 - Teaspoons Worcestershire sauce
1/2 - Cup dry red wine (may use 1/2 cup additional broth)

Instructions:

Trim excess fat and any bones from the roast. Cut the roast in half. Empty 1 pouch of soup mix into the bottom of a crock pot. Add 1 can of broth, Worcestershire sauce and mix. Place the 2 pieces of roast on edge and side by side in the crock pot. Add the other pouch of soup mix and the wine. Cook on high heat for approximately 5 hours (2 hours per pound of beef); then reduce heat to low and let simmer for an additional hour. Serve hot and in chunks. Spoon the liquids, as a gravy, over the serving.
Serves 4 to 6

Category of Recipe: | Beef

Name of Recipe: | Bacon Wrapped Filet Mignon with Hollandaise Sauce

Recipe Color Code: | Red

Ingredients:

4 - Filets mignons, about 1 1/2 pounds
1/2 - Teaspoon salt, divided
1/2 - Teaspoon ground black pepper, divided
8 - Slices bacon
1 - Tablespoon plus 1/2 cup butter, divided
12 - Ounces fresh mushrooms, quartered
3 - Egg yolks
1 - Tablespoon lemon juice
1 - Tablespoon fresh parsley, chopped

Instructions:

Season beef with 1/4 teaspoon salt and 1/4 teaspoon pepper. Wrap 2 slices of bacon in criss-cross fashion around each filet. In skillet, melt 1 tablespoon butter over medium heat. Cook beef and mushrooms until golden, about 9 minutes per side for medium, turning beef on Its side to brown and stirring mushrooms occasionally. Transfer beef and mushrooms to a serving platter. Meanwhile, place remaining butter in a small glass bowl. Cover with vented plastic wrap. Cook in microwave on high for 45 seconds or until melted; set aside. In a pot over low heat combine egg yolks, lemon juice and 5 tablespoons water. Cook, whisking constantly, until mixture is creamy and coats back of spoon, about 8 minutes. Quickly transfer yolk mixture to blender; add remaining salt and pepper. With blender on high, add remaining melted butter in a steady stream until combined and thickened, about 30 seconds. Spoon sauce over beef. Sprinkle with parsley.
Serves 4

Category of Recipe: | Beef

Name of Recipe: | Taco Boat

Recipe Color Code: | Red

Ingredients:

1 - Pound lean ground beef
1 - Medium green pepper, finely chopped
1 - Medium onion, finely chopped
1 - Head iceberg lettuce
2 - Tablespoons chili powder
3/4 - Teaspoon cumin
1/2 - Teaspoon salt
1 - Teaspoon garlic powder
2 - Tablespoons canola oil
1 - 8 ounce container sour cream
3/4 - Cup sliced black olives
1/2 - Cup sliced jalapeno peppers (optional)
1 - Cup Kraft finely shredded "Mexican Four Cheese"
1 - Cup salsa, no sugar or corn syrup added

Instructions:

Sauté the onion and pepper in canola oil until done. Remove from skillet and set aside. Cook the ground beef until 3/4 done. Add the chili powder, salt, garlic powder, and cumin. Stir into beef and finish cooking until done. Stir occasionally to prevent burning. Add the cooked onions and peppers to the mixture, stir, and heat thoroughly. Remove the core and loose leaves from the head of lettuce. Beginning at the core end, cut the head of lettuce into halves. Remove the small center section from both halves, leaving the stacked "boats" of lettuce. Remove a "boat" from the lettuce. This will be a thickness of 3 to 5 leaves. Place 3 to 5 tablespoons of the cooked beef mixture into the lettuce "boat." Top with the shredded cheese, then sour cream, salsa, black olives, and jalapeno peppers as desired.
Serves 2 to 3

Category of Recipe: Beef

Name of Recipe: Poor Boy Filets

Recipe Color Code: Red

Ingredients:

1 - Pound ground beef
1 - Teaspoon Worcestershire sauce
1/4 - Teaspoon garlic powder
1 - Teaspoon margarine
1 - Teaspoon salt
4 - Slices bacon

Instructions:

Preheat broiler. Combine ground beef, Worcestershire sauce, garlic powder, margarine, salt, and pepper; mix well. Shape into 4 patties and wrap each patty with a slice of bacon, fastening with wooden toothpicks. Place patties on broiler rack and broil 1 minute; turn and broil 1 minute longer. Turn broiler off and allow patties to stay in broiler 30 minutes. Meat will be very juicy. Serve with sautéed mushrooms desired.
Serves 4

Category of Recipe: Beef

Name of Recipe: London Broil

Recipe Color Code: Red

Ingredients:

1 - 1 1/2 - Pounds flank steak
1/3 - Cup canola oil
1 - Tablespoon red wine vinegar
2 - Cloves garlic, minced
1/2 - Teaspoon salt
1/4 - Teaspoon ground black pepper

Instructions:

Trim excess fat from steak; score steak on both sides in one and one half inch squares. Place steak in a deep bowl. Combine oil, vinegar, and garlic; pour over meat and marinate 3 hours in refrigerator, turning once after 1/12 hours. Preheat oven broiler. Remove steak from marinade and place on a lightly greased rack in broiler pan. Broil 4 inches from heat for 5 minutes. Sprinkle with half of the salt and pepper. Turn steak over, sprinkle on other half of salt and pepper. Broil for an additional 5 minutes. To serve, slice across the grain into thin slices.
Serves 4 to 6

Category of Recipe:	Beef

Name of Recipe:	Onion Fried Steak

Recipe Color Code:	Red

Ingredients:

2 - 8 to 12 ounce rib eye steaks
1/2 - Teaspoon salt
1/4 - Cup chopped green onions
1/4 - Cup margarine

Instructions:

Sprinkle both sides of steaks with salt; set aside. In a large skillet, melt the margarine over low heat. Sauté the 1/4 cup green onions until crisp-tender. Remove onions from skillet and set aside. Add steaks to the skillet and cook over medium heat for 8 minutes. Turn steaks and continue cooking for an additional 8 minutes, or until the steaks reach desired degree of doneness. Remove the steaks to serving platter or individual plates; sprinkle with the cooked green onions.
Serves 2

Category of Recipe: | Beef

Name of Recipe: | Cracked Pepper Steak

Recipe Color Code: | Red

Ingredients:

2 - 8 to 12 ounce rib eye steaks
1/4 - Teaspoon garlic powder
1/2 - Teaspoon salt
1/4 - Cup green onions, chopped
1/4 - Cup margarine, melted
1 - Teaspoon cracked black pepper, divided

Instructions:

Sprinkle both sides of the steaks with garlic powder and salt; set aside. In a large skillet (large enough for the two steaks), melt the margarine over low heat. Sauté the 1/4 cup of green onions over medium-low heat until crisp-tender. Remove onions from skillet and set aside. Sprinkle 1/2 teaspoon pepper in the skillet; add steaks and cook over medium heat for approximately 8 minutes. Sprinkle remaining 1/2 teaspoon pepper over the top of the steaks; turn and continue cooking for an additional 8 minutes or until the steaks have reached a desired degree of doneness. Remove the steaks to a serving platter, or individual plates, and sprinkle with the cooked onions.
Serves 2

Category of Recipe: | Beef

Name of Recipe: | Steak Diane Flambé

Recipe Color Code: | Red

Ingredients:

2 - 8 ounce rib eye steaks
1/2 - Cup sliced fresh mushrooms
1/4 - Cup chopped green onions
2 - Tablespoons butter or margarine, melted
2 - Tablespoons brandy
1 - Tablespoon Worcestershire sauce
1/2 - Teaspoon dry mustard
1/8 - Teaspoon salt
1/8 - Teaspoon ground black pepper

Instructions:

Place steaks between 2 pieces of waxed paper; pound with meat mallet to flatten slightly. In a large skillet, melt butter over medium-low heat. Sauté mushrooms and green onions in the melted butter until tender. Push mushroom mixture to one side of the skillet. Add steaks, cook until done, browning on both sides; remove from heat. Over medium-low heat, heat brandy in a long-handled sauce pan just long enough to produce fumes (do not boil). Remove brandy from heat, ignite, and pour over steaks. When flames die down, remove steaks from skillet and place them on a serving platter. Add Worcestershire sauce, dry mustard, salt, and black pepper to the mushroom mixture in skillet; blend well, and cook 1 minute. Evenly spoon mushroom mixture over top of steaks.
Serves 2

Category of Recipe: | Beef

Name of Recipe: | Mexican Steak

Recipe Color Code: | Red

Ingredients:

1 1/4 - Pounds boneless round steak
2 - Tablespoons butter or margarine, melted
1 - 4 ounce can chopped green chilies, drained
1 - 8 ounce jar taco sauce
1/2 - Cup (2 ounces) shredded Monterey Jack cheese

Instructions:

Trim excess fat from steak. Cut steak into 4 pieces and pound to 1/4 inch thickness using a meat mallet. Preheat oven to 350 degrees. In a large skillet and over medium- low heat, melt the butter. In the melted butter, brown the steaks on both sides. Place the browned steaks in a lightly greased shallow 2 quart casserole dish. Top the steaks with green chilies and taco sauce. Cover and bake at 350 degrees for 40 minutes. Sprinkle with shredded cheese and bake uncovered, an additional 5 minutes.
Serves 4

Category of Recipe: | Beef

Name of Recipe: | Grecian Skillet Rib Eye Steak

Recipe Color Code: | Red

Ingredients:

2 - Well trimmed beef rib eye steaks, about 3/4 inch thick
1 - Tablespoon olive oil
1 - Tablespoon fresh lemon juice
2 - Tablespoons crumbled feta cheese
1 - Tablespoon chopped, pitted ripe olives
Below seasonings:
   1 1/2 - Teaspoon garlic powder
   1 1/2 - Teaspoon dried basil leaves, crushed
   1 1/2 - Teaspoon dried oregano leaves, crushed
   1/2 - Teaspoon salt
   1/4 - Teaspoon ground black pepper

Instructions:

Combine seasoning ingredients; press into both sides of beef steaks. In a large non-stick skillet, heat olive oil over medium heat until hot. Place steaks in skillet; cook approximately 10 to 14 minutes for medium-rare to medium doneness, turning once. Cook longer for done, etc., to taste. Sprinkle with lemon juice. To serve, sprinkle cheese and olives over steaks.
Serves 2

Category of Recipe: | Beef

Name of Recipe: | Spaghetti (squash) with Meat Sauce

Recipe Color Code: | Red

Ingredients:

1 – 2 ½ to 3 pound whole spaghetti squash
1 – pound ground chuck
1 – medium onion, chopped (about 1 cup)
1 – medium green pepper, chopped (about 1 cup)
2 – garlic cloves, minced
1 – 14 ½ ounce can diced tomatoes, undrained
1 – 6 ounce can tomato sauce
2 – tablespoons tomato paste
1 ½ - teaspoons dried Italian seasoning, crushed
½ - teaspoon ground black pepper
¼ - cup shredded Parmesan cheese (about 1 ounce)

Instructions:

Prick the squash in 8 to 12 places, about evenly spaced, with a sharp knife to let steam escape while cooking. Place squash in a microwave baking dish and microwave on high power about 12 minutes. Let stand at least 5 minutes. Half squash lengthwise and remove seeds. Use a fork to shred out and separate the pulp into strands. Keep strands warm for serving later.

Prepare the sauce large sauce pan by cooking the ground beef, onion, garlic, and green pepper until the meat is done. Drain off the fat. Add undrained diced tomatoes, tomato sauce, tomato paste, Italian seasoning, and black pepper. Bring sauce to boil, reduce heat and simmer uncovered for 15 minutes, occasionally stirring to prevent scorching. Place a serving of spaghetti squash on a dinner plate and ladle on a desired about of meat sauce. Sprinkle each serving with Parmesan cheese in the amount of choice.
Serves 4
Note: Squash and sauce may be cooked at same time.

Category of Recipe: | Beef

Name of Recipe: | Barbecued Brisket

Recipe Color Code: | Red

Ingredients:

1 – 4 to 5 pounds beef brisket
½ - teaspoon celery salt
¼ - teaspoon garlic powder
¼ – teaspoon onion powder
2 – Tablespoons liquid smoke
1/3 – cup Worcestershire Sauce
¾ - cup commercial prepared barbeque sauce

Instructions:

Place brisket in a shallow baking dish. Sprinkle beef with celery salt, garlic powder and onion powder. Mix the liquid smoke and Worcestershire sauce and pour mixture over the beef. Cover with aluminum foil and refrigerate for a minimum of 8 hours, turning once after 4 hours. Preheat oven to 300 degrees. Cover brisket and bake at 300 degrees for 4 hours or until tender. Pour off liquid, reserving ½ cup. Combine the reserved liquid with the barbecue sauce, mixing well. Pour sauce over beef and bake, uncovered, an additional 30 minutes. To serve, slice across the grain into thin slices.
Serves 8 to 10

Note: Keep in the refrigerator and slice as desired.

Category of Recipe: | Beef

Name of Recipe: | Stuffed Green Peppers

Recipe Color Code: | Red

Ingredients:

4 - Large green peppers
1 1/4 - Pound ground beef
1 - Medium onion, chopped
1 - 8 ounce can tomato sauce
2 - Tablespoons tomato paste
2 - Teaspoons chili powder
1/2 - Teaspoon salt
1/2 - Cup (2 ounces) shredded cheddar cheese

Instructions:

Cut off tops of green peppers; remove centers and discard. Cook peppers 5 minutes in boiling water; drain peppers and set aside. Pre-heat oven to 350 degrees. Cook ground beef and onion in a large deep skillet until meat is browned, stirring to crumble meat; drain well. Stir in tomato sauce, tomato paste, chili powder, and salt. Stuff peppers with meat mixture, and place in a baking dish that has been sprayed with Pam cooking spray. Bake at 350 degrees for 15 minutes. Sprinkle tops of peppers with cheese; bake an additional 5 minutes.
Serves 4

Category of Recipe: | Casserole

Name of Recipe: | Pizza Casserole

Recipe Color Code: | Red

Ingredients:

1 - Pound lean ground beef
1 - Cup crushed tomatoes with added puree
2 - Tablespoons olive oil
1/2 - Cup sliced mushrooms
1/2 - Cup green bell pepper, chopped
1 - Teaspoon salt
1 - Teaspoon oregano
1/2 - Teaspoon basil
1/2 - Teaspoon thyme
8 - Ounces shredded mozzarella cheese
2 - Ounces shredded Parmesan cheese

Instructions:

Heat oil in a skillet on medium heat. Sauté onions, peppers, mushrooms, and seasonings until tender, stirring frequently to prevent scorching. Set aside. Cook the ground beef until done, stirring to break into small pieces. Add the sautéed vegetables to the cooked meat and stir. Add the tomatoes and stir. Divide in half. Pre-heat oven to 350 degrees. Spray an 8 inch x 10 inch baking dish with a non-stick cooking spray. Put half of the cooked meat mixture in the baking dish. Cover with 1/2 of the mozzarella cheese. Put the other half of the cooked meat mixture over the cheese. Cover with the other half of the mozzarella cheese. Cover mozzarella cheese with the Parmesan cheese. Bake at 350 degrees for 35 minutes.
Serves 6

Category of Recipe: Casserole

Name of Recipe: Broccoli and Cauliflower Casserole

Recipe Color Code: Yellow

Ingredients:

1 - 16 ounce package broccoli florets, thawed and well drained
1 - 16 ounce package cauliflower, thawed and drained
1 - Cup canola oil mayonnaise
3 - Tablespoons Dijon mustard
1/2 - Teaspoon salt
1/2 - Cup grated cheddar cheese

Instructions:

Preheat oven to 375 degrees. Combine all ingredients, except the cheese, in a large bowl. Mix until all the vegetables are well coated. Spray a 1 1/2 quart baking dish with a non-stick cooking spray and pour the mixture into the dish. Sprinkle the vegetable mixture with the cheddar cheese. Bake for about 30 minutes until the cheese is a golden brown. Serve while hot.
Serves 6

Category of Recipe: | Casserole |

Name of Recipe: | Squash Casserole |

Recipe Color Code: | Red |

Ingredients:

8 – Tablespoons olive oil, divided
1 – large onion, chopped
3 – stalks celery, chopped
1 – 8 ounce package fresh sliced mushrooms
½ - cup mayonnaise
1 – 8 ounce container sour cream
2 – large eggs, beaten
2 – cups Colby jack shredded cheese
Salt to taste
Pepper to taste
8 – cups raw fresh yellow squash, cut into bite size
pieces

Instructions:

Pre-heat oven to 350 degrees. Heat 4 tablespoons olive oil in a large skillet over medium heat. Sauté the onion and celery for approximately 5 minutes or until tender. Add the mushrooms and sauté for an additional 10 minutes or until the vegetables are tender. Place the sautéed mixture in a large bowl to cool. In the same skillet, heat the other 4 tablespoons olive oil. Add the squash, salt and pepper. Sauté the squash until tender but still firm. Add the cooked squash to the large bowl that contains the other cooked mixture. To the same large bowl, add the mayonnaise, sour cream, beaten eggs, and cheese. Mix all ingredients well. Spray a large baking dish with non-stick cooking spray. Pour the mixture into the baking dish, even out, and bake at 350 degrees for 40 minutes. Remove from oven, let stand for 5 minutes, then serve.
Serves 6 to 8

Category of Recipe: | Casserole

Name of Recipe: | Crustless Quiche

Recipe Color Code: | Red

Ingredients:

½ - pound bacon, crispy fried and crumbled
1 – cup shredded Swiss cheese
1/3 – cup minced onion
4 – eggs
2 – cups light cream
¾ - teaspoon salt
1/8 – teaspoon ground black pepper
½ - packet artificial sweetener
1 – package spinach, frozen, drained

Instructions:

Preheat oven to 425 degrees. Spray quiche dish with Pam. Sprinkle cheese, bacon and onion on the bottom of dish. Beat remaining ingredients until blended and pour over bacon mixture. Cover edge with aluminum foil to prevent browning. Bake 15 minutes. Reduce oven temperature to 300 degrees and bake 35 additional minutes. Remove foil for the last 15 minutes. Let stand 10 minutes before slicing.
Serves 4 to 6

Category of Recipe: | Casserole

Name of Recipe: | Breakfast Casserole

Recipe Color Code: | Red

Ingredients:

7 - Large, or jumbo, eggs
3/4 - Cup sour cream
1 - Teaspoon salt
1/2 - Teaspoon ground black pepper
8 – Approximately 3/8" sausage patties, cooked
    (may substitute ham or bacon)
3/4 - Cup shredded Monterey Jack cheese
3/4 - Cup shredded cheddar cheese
1 – Cup salsa, drained
Parsley, or other garnish as desired

Instructions:

Pre-heat oven to 325 degrees. While sausage, bacon or ham is cooking, place eggs, sour cream, salsa, salt, pepper, and both cheeses in a large mixing bowl. Mix well with wire whisk. Spray a 9" round by 2" deep (or large rectangular) baking dish with a non-stick spray. Pour the egg, cream, salsa, and cheese mixture into the baking dish. Evenly distribute the cooked sausage patties, ham or bacon over the mixture. Bake at 325 degrees for 35 minutes, or, until a knife inserted near the center comes out clean. Remove from oven and let stand 5 minutes before slicing into approximately 8 individual servings. Place individual serving on a plate. Garnish serving as desired.
Serves 6 to 8

Note: Refrigerate any remaining servings. To re-heat a serving, wrap with damp paper towel and microwave on high for 1 minute. A great breakfast for those on the run.

Category of Recipe: | Dessert

Name of Recipe: | Ice Cream

Recipe Color Code: | Red

Ingredients:

5 - Egg yolks
3 - Teaspoons vanilla extract
8 - Teaspoons equivalents sugar substitute
1/4 - Cup water
2 - Cups heavy whipping cream (whipped)

Instructions:

Place yolks, vanilla extract, sugar substitute, and water in blender and blend at medium speed for 30 seconds. Fold yolk mixture into whipped cream. Blend well being careful not to break down the whipped cream. Empty into refrigerator tray, freeze for two hours.
Serves 4

Category of Recipe: | Dessert

Name of Recipe: | Old-Fashion Baked Custard

Recipe Color Code: | Red

Ingredients:

2 – cups heavy cream
1- teaspoon vanilla extract
2 – eggs
2 – egg yolks
¼ - teaspoon salt
6 – packets artificial sweetener

Instructions:

Place the cream and vanilla in a saucepan and mix. Cook the mixture over medium heat just until it begins to steam. Using a mixing bowl, combine the eggs, egg yolks, salt, and artificial sweetener. Beat the mixture with a whisk or an electric mixer until it is a pale yellow in color and is fairly thick. Preheat oven to 300 degrees and place a kettle of water on high heat to boil (first, read the rest of this recipe to understand the use of the hot water). Gradually add the cream to the egg mixture, stirring constantly while adding. Pour, and evenly distribute, the cream and egg mixture into six 6-ounce custard cups (or a large bowl may be used instead of the custard cups). Place the custard cups (or bowl) in a baking pan with sides. Pour the hot water into the baking pan to within about 1 inch to the top of the cups (or bowl). Bake the cups for about 30 minutes (a little longer if using a bowl). Serve warm, at room temperature, or cold within a day.
Serves 6

Category of Recipe: | Dessert

Name of Recipe: | Sugar Free Pudding

Recipe Color Code: | Red

Ingredients:

1 – package instant sugar free Jell-O (flavor of choice)
2 – cups whipping cream

Instructions:

Mix ingredients together using hand mixer. Cover with saran wrap and refrigerate.
Serves 2

Note: This is a very simple recipe for a great tasting treat

Category of Recipe:	Grains and Beans
Name of Recipe:	Oatmeal
Recipe Color Code:	Green

Ingredients:

1/3 - "Heaping" cup **rolled** oats (may be purchased in
  bulk at most health food stores
3/4 - Cup water
1/4 - Teaspoon salt (optional)
2 - Packages artificial sweetener (optional)
1/2 - Cup skimmed milk

Instructions:

Using a microwaveable bowl that will hold a minimum of
2 cups, add water to the oats and salt as desired. Stir.
Microwave on high for 2 1/2 minutes. Stir. Microwave
on high for an additional 35 seconds. Stir. Add
sweetener to taste. Stir. Add milk to taste.
Serves 1

Note: You will notice that this oatmeal has a "nutty"
flavor as compared to the "wall paste" taste of regular
oatmeal.

Category of Recipe: Grains and Beans

Name of Recipe: Pinto Beans with Ham

Recipe Color Code: Red

Ingredients:

1 – pound package pinto beans
2 – ham hocks
2 – teaspoons salt
½ - teaspoon ground black pepper
Water

Instructions:

Place dried pinto beans in a large mixing bowl or large pan. Cover with water to above 2 inches above the top of the beans. Soak overnight. Rinse beans in a colander, discarding the water. Placed the rinsed beans in a large crock pot. Add the ham hocks, salt and black pepper. Cover the mixture with water to approximately 2 ½ inches over the top of the beans. Cook in the crock pot on high heat for approximately 6 hours or until the beans are tender. Serve in individual bowls.
Serves 4 to 6

Note: This is a great southern dish that is commonly served in lieu of soup on a chilly day.

Category of Recipe: | Pork

Name of Recipe: | Pork Roast

Recipe Color Code: | Red

Ingredients:

1 – 3 to 4 pound pork loin
1 – teaspoon dried rosemary
¼ - teaspoon cayenne pepper (optional)
1 – clove garlic, minced
1 ½ - cups dry white wine
1 – tablespoon butter
2 – teaspoons salt
½ - teaspoon ground black pepper.

Instructions:

Preheat oven to 450 degrees. Mix the salt, black pepper, cayenne, rosemary, and garlic. Rub the mixture in all over the roast. Place the rubbed loin in a roasting pan and put in the oven (use a rack in the pan if the loin is boneless). Roast at the 450 degrees for 15 minutes. Open the oven door and pour ½ cup of the wine over the roast. Close the oven door and reduce the heat to 325 degrees. Continue cooking, adding ¼ cup of the wine each 15 minutes. After reducing the heat, roast for about 1 ½ hours or until the interior of the roast reaches 150 degrees. When done, remove the roast to a platter. Place the pan over a burner set at medium-high heat. Reduce the liquid to about ¼ cup, scraping the bottom of the pan to release any brown bits. When the sauce has reduced some, stir in the butter. Slice the roast and serve with some of the sauce drizzled over each serving. Serves 6 to 8

Category of Recipe:	Pork
Name of Recipe:	Dijon Pork Chops
Recipe Color Code:	Red

Ingredients:

4 - Pork chops, cut approximately 1/2 inch thick
3 - Tablespoons Dijon mustard
2 - Tablespoons Italian salad dressing (do not use low-fat)
1/4 - Teaspoon ground black pepper
1/4 - Teaspoon salt
1 - Medium onion, sliced

Instructions:

In a small bowl, combine mustard, Italian dressing, salt and pepper. Set aside. Spray a 10 inch skillet with a non-stick cooking spray. Preheat the skillet over medium heat. Add the pork chops and brown on both sides. Remove the chops from skillet. Add onion to skillet. Cook and stir over medium heat for 3 minutes. Push the onion aside and return the chops to the skillet. Spread the mustard mixture over the pork chops. Cover and cook over medium-low heat for 15 minutes or until chops are no longer pink inside. Place cooked chops and plate, cover with the onion mixture, and serve.
Serves 4

Category of Recipe: | Pork

Name of Recipe: | Crusted Pork Chops

Recipe Color Code: | Red

Ingredients:

4 - Pork loin rib chops
1 - Fresh lemon
1/4 - Cup olive oil
2 - Teaspoon dried rosemary
2 - Teaspoon dried thyme
1 - Clove garlic, minced
3/4 - Teaspoon salt
1/2 - Teaspoon ground black pepper
12 - Ounces fresh mushrooms, sliced
1 - Tablespoon butter
1 - Cup chicken broth

Instructions:

Grate 1 teaspoon of peel from lemon. Place grated lemon peel, 2 tablespoons lemon juice, olive oil, rosemary, thyme, garlic, 1/2 teaspoon salt and 1/4 teaspoon pepper in a zip-top bag. Add pork chops and toss to coat. Seal and marinate in refrigerator at least 1 hour, turning occasionally to coat the chops. Remove chops from bag. Heat skillet over medium-high. Add chops and cook until the meat is no longer pink (this usually takes about 4 minutes per side). Remove cooked chops and place on a serving platter; keep warm. In same skillet, melt butter over medium heat. Add mushrooms and cook about 5 minutes until golden. Add remaining ingredients to skillet. Bring to a boil then simmer 2 to 3 minutes until thickened. Serve mushroom gravy over the pork chops.
Serves 4

Category of Recipe: | Pork

Name of Recipe: | Cuban Style Roast Pork

Recipe Color Code: | Red

Ingredients:

1 - Fresh ham, about 8 pounds
6 - Cloves garlic, minced
1 - Tablespoon salt
1 - Bay leaf
2 - Teaspoons dried oregano
1 - Teaspoon dried thyme
1 - Teaspoon ground cumin
1 - Teaspoon ground black pepper
1/4 - Cup olive oil
1/2 - Cup orange juice
1/2 - Cup lime juice
2 - Large onions, sliced into thin rings

Instructions:

Trim excess fat from the ham. Make shallow cuts in a criss-cross fashion all over the ham (forming about 1/2 inch squares). Using a food processor, mix salt and garlic together. Add bay leaf, oregano, thyme and pepper. Process into a thick paste. Add orange juice, lime juice and olive oil. Mix well. Rub mixture well into the cuts made on ham. Place 1/2 the onions in a non-corrosive container. Place the ham on the onions and cover the ham with the remaining onions. Cover with plastic wrap and refrigerate overnight (turn once about every 4 hours). Preheat oven to 350 degrees. Drain the ham, reserving marinade. Pat the ham dry with paper towels. Place ham in a lightly oiled non-corrosive roasting pan. Roast 1 hour, turning every 15 minutes to brown all sides. Pour the reserved marinade and onions over ham roast. Tent with foil, reduce heat to 325 degrees and roast for 2 hours or until the center of ham reaches at least 180 degrees; or until done. Baste about every 30 minutes while cooking.
Serves 10

Category of Recipe: | Poultry

Name of Recipe: | Egg Salad

Recipe Color Code: | Red

Ingredients:

8 - Eggs, hard boiled
1 - Teaspoon Dijon mustard
2 - Tablespoon chopped pickles (dill or sweet of choice)
3/4 - Cup canola oil mayonnaise
Salt to taste
Pepper to taste

Instructions:

Coarsely chop the eggs. Fold the eggs into all the other ingredients. Refrigerate and serve on a bed of lettuce.
Serves 4

Category of Recipe: Poultry

Name of Recipe: Poached Eggs

Recipe Color Code: Red

Ingredients:

1 1/2 - Quarts water
2 - Cups vinegar
8 - Large eggs

Instructions:

In a large sauce pan, combine water and vinegar. Bring to boil. Crack the eggs one at a time and gently drop them into the boiling water. Be careful not to break the yolks. Simmer for 4 minutes, moving eggs several times with a spoon to cook them thoroughly. When the eggs are cooked to a firm consistency, remove them from the water with a slotted spoon and place in a pan filled with cold water until served.
Serves 4 to 6

Category of Recipe: Poultry

Name of Recipe: Chicken Monterey

Recipe Color Code: Red

Ingredients:

4 - Boneless and skinless chicken breast halves
3 - Tablespoons olive oil
1 - Teaspoon onion powder
1 - Teaspoon oregano
1/2 - Teaspoon thyme
1/2 - Teaspoon ground black pepper
1/2 - Teaspoon salt
1 - Medium onion, evenly sliced into about 1/4" slices
4 - Slices bacon, cooked
4 - Slices Monterey Jack cheese

Instructions:

Heat olive oil on medium heat in a large deep skillet that has a lid. While oil is heating, pat chicken breast dry with paper towels. Mix the onion powder, oregano, thyme, black pepper, and salt together and sprinkle both sides of the chicken with the mixture. Place chicken breast in heated oil, cover with lid, and cook until about 1/2 done. Turn the chicken over and finish cooking uncovered, until chicken is done. On each breast half, place a large slice of onion, one strip of the cooked bacon, and top these with the Monterey Jack cheese. Turn off heat and let set until cheese is melted.
Serves 4

Category of Recipe:	Poultry
Name of Recipe:	Chicken with Lemon Basil Sauce
Recipe Color Code:	Red

Ingredients:

3 - Tablespoons olive oil
4 - Chicken breast halves, boneless and skinless
3 - Tablespoons fresh lemon juice
3 - Cloves garlic, minced
1 - Cup canned low salt chicken broth
1 - Tablespoon dried basil
1 - Teaspoon (packed) grated lemon peel

Instructions:

Heat olive oil in heavy large skillet over medium high heat. Sprinkle chicken with salt and pepper. Add chicken to skillet and sauté until brown and cooked through, about 5 minutes per side uncovered; and, 4 minutes on each side covered. Transfer chicken to platter; tent with aluminum foil. Add lemon juice, garlic and lemon peel to same skillet. Stir over medium high heat until fragrant, about 30 seconds. Add chicken broth; boil until reduced to sauce consistency, about 8 minutes. Stir frequently. Mix basil into sauce. Season to taste with salt and pepper. Spoon sauce over chicken and serve.
Serves 4

Category of Recipe: | Poultry |

Name of Recipe: | Chicken Cordon Blue |

Recipe Color Code: | Red |

Ingredients:

4 - Chicken breast halves, boneless and skinless
4 - Slices smoked ham, thinly sliced
4 - Slices Swiss cheese
4 - Slices bacon

Instructions:

Pre-heat oven to 350 degrees. Using a chopping block covered with waxed paper and using a meat mallet, pound the chicken breast to approximately 1/4 inch thick. Pre-cook bacon until about 75% done. Place on slice of ham and one slice of cheese on each breast half. Roll into a roll and wrap diagonally with one slice bacon. Use wood tooth picks to hold each end of the bacon in place. Spray a 9 inch x 12 inch baking dish with non-stick cooking spray. Lay rolled breast halves in baking dish and lightly sprinkle with any spice or herb of choice, such as salt, pepper, basil, tetragon, etc. Bake at 350 degrees for 50 minutes.
Serves 4

Note: This is a great dish!

Category of Recipe: Poultry

Name of Recipe: Plain Omelet

Recipe Color Code: Red

Ingredients:

2 - Eggs
1/8 - Teaspoon salt
Dash of black pepper
1 - Tablespoon water
1 - Tablespoon margarine
Omelet filling of choice (cheese, ham, bacon, onion, etc.)

Instructions:

Combine eggs, salt, pepper, and water; whisk egg mixture just until blended. Heat a 6" or *" omelet pan or heavy skillet over medium heat until hot enough to sizzle a drop of water. Add margarine to the skillet, and rotate pan to coat bottom evenly. Pour egg mixture into the skillet. As mixture starts to cook, gently lift edges of omelet with a spatula, and tilt pan to uncooked portion flows underneath. Sprinkle half of the omelet with one or more of the following fillings of choice: 2 slices bacon cooked and crumbled, 2 tablespoons sautéed mushroom slices, 2 tablespoons shredded cheese of choice, 2 tablespoons diced cooked ham. For a Spanish omelet, add 2 tablespoons picante sauce. Fold omelet in half, and transfer to plate.
Serves 1

Category of Recipe: | Poultry

Name of Recipe: | Cajun Chicken

Recipe Color Code: | Red

Ingredients:

4 - Boneless and skinless chicken breast halves
1 - 6 ounce can Hot and Spicy V-8 juice
2 - Tablespoons Cajun spice of choice

Instructions:

Pre-heat oven to 350 degrees. Spray a 9" x 13" baking dish with non-stick cooking spray. Place chicken in baking dish. Pour the V-8 juice over chicken and sprinkle with Cajun spice. Bake at 350 degrees for 40 minutes.
Serves 4

Category of Recipe: | Poultry

Name of Recipe: | Chicken in Wine and Olive Sauce

Recipe Color Code: | Red

Ingredients:

4 - Boneless and skinless chicken breast halves
2 - Tablespoons olive oil
1/2 - Teaspoon salt
1/4 - Teaspoon ground black pepper
1 - Large onion, thinly sliced
3/4 - Cup dry white wine
1/2 - Cup stuffed green olives, sliced
1/2 - Teaspoon thyme
1 - Teaspoon basil
1 - Tablespoon water

Instructions:

In a non-stick skillet, heat olive oil over medium-high heat. Add chicken. Sprinkle with the salt and pepper. Cook until lightly browned on both sides, turning once or twice. Remove chicken from skillet and place on plate. Using same skillet, cook onion in the pan drippings until golden brown, stirring frequently to prevent burning. Add wine, olives, thyme, and basil. Stir and return the browned chicken, along with the juices from the plate, to the skillet. Reduce heat to low, cover and simmer for 20 to 25 minutes. (Add more wine if pan becomes too dry during cooking. When done, remove cooked chicken to individually warmed plates for serving. Spoon sauce from pan over individual servings of chicken as desired. Serves 4

Category of Recipe: | Poultry

Name of Recipe: | Chicken Cacciatore

Recipe Color Code: | Red

Ingredients:

1 - Large onion, thinly sliced
1 1/2 - Pounds chicken breast halves, skinned and
   boneless
2 - 6 ounce cans tomato paste
8 - Ounces fresh sliced mushrooms
1/2 - Teaspoon salt
1/4 - Teaspoon ground black pepper
2 - Garlic cloves, minced
1 - Teaspoon oregano
1/2 - Teaspoon basil
1 - Bay leaf
1/4 - Cup dry white wine
1/4 - Chicken broth

Instructions:

Put the sliced onion in bottom of crock pot. Add chicken.
Stir together tomato paste, mushrooms, salt, pepper,
garlic, herbs, white wine and water. Spread over the
chicken. Cover; cook on high for 3 1/2 hours, or until
chicken is done and tender. Place chicken on serving
plates and spoon liquid mixture over each piece.
Serves 4

Category of Recipe: Poultry

Name of Recipe: Hunter's Style Chicken

Recipe Color Code: Red

Ingredients:

4 - Chicken breast halves, boneless and skinless
6 - Tablespoons olive oil, divided
1 - Large onion, chopped
1 - Green pepper, chopped
1/2 - Teaspoon basil
2 - Cloves garlic, minced
1/2 - Teaspoon salt
1/2 - Teaspoon ground black pepper
1 - 10 ounce can RO-TEL brand diced tomatoes with
    chilies
1/2 - Teaspoon tarragon
1/2 - Cup sliced and prepared mushrooms (1small jar)
Grated Parmesan cheese for topping (optional)

Instructions:

In a large skillet, sauté onion and pepper in 3 tablespoons olive oil until tender (do not brown). Add garlic, basil, salt, and black pepper. Stir. Cover and sauté about 3 more minutes, stirring frequently. Remove mixture from skillet and set aside. Using same skillet, cook chicken in 3 tablespoons of olive oil over medium heat until done and evenly brown on all sides. Once the chicken is cooked and browned, add the onion and pepper mixture. Also add the undrained RO-TEL tomatoes and the mushrooms. Stir. Cover and cook on medium heat for approximately 5 minutes. Turn the chick, stir, and cook an additional 3 minutes until the mixture is evenly heated. Remove chicken to serving dish and spoon onion, pepper, and tomato mixture over the chicken. Sprinkle with grated cheese as desired. Serves 4

Category of Recipe: Poultry

Name of Recipe: Cracked Pepper Fried Chicken with Green Onions

Recipe Color Code: Red

Ingredients:

4 - Chicken breast halves, skinless and boneless
1/4 - Teaspoon garlic powder
1/2 - Teaspoon salt
1/2 - Cup green onions, chopped
1/4 - Cup margarine, melted
2 - Tablespoons canola oil
1 - Teaspoon cracked black pepper, divided

Instructions:

Sprinkle both sides of the chicken breast halves with garlic powder and salt; set aside. In a large skillet with lid (large enough for the 4 chicken breast halves), melt the margarine over medium-low heat. Sauté the 1/4 cup of green onions uncovered until crisp tender. Remove onions from skillet and set aside. Add canola oil to the skillet and heat over medium heat. Sprinkle 1/2 teaspoon pepper in the skillet, add chicken, cover, and cook over medium heat for 7 minutes or until 1/2 done. Sprinkle remaining 1/2 teaspoon pepper over the top of the chicken, turn, cov3er, and continue cooking for an additional 7 minutes or until chicken is completely done. Remove the lid and brown the chicken on both sides. Remove chicken to serving platter and sprinkle with the cooked onions.
Serves 4

Category of Recipe: | Poultry

Name of Recipe: | Crock Pot Chicken Cacciatore

Recipe Color Code: | Red

Ingredients:

1 - Large onion, thinly sliced
1 1/2 - Pounds chicken breast halves, skinned and
          boneless
2 - 6 ounce cans tomato paste
8 - Ounces fresh sliced mushrooms
1/2 - Teaspoon salt
1/4 - Teaspoon ground black pepper
2 - Garlic cloves, minced
1 - Teaspoon oregano
1/2 - Teaspoon basil
1 - Bay leaf
1/4 - Cup dry white wine
1/4 - Chicken broth

Instructions:

Place the sliced onion in bottom of crock pot. Add chicken. Stir together tomato paste, mushrooms, salt, pepper, garlic, herbs, white wine and water. Spread over the chicken. Cover and cook on high for 3 1/2 hours, or until chicken is done and tender. Place chicken on serving plates and spoon liquid mixture over each piece. Serves 4

Category of Recipe: | Poultry

Name of Recipe: | Easy Chicken Stir Fry

Recipe Color Code: | Red

Ingredients:

1 - 16 ounce package Bird's Eye brand "Pepper Stir Fry"
(red, yellow, and green peppers, plus onions.)
1 - 1 pound package Green Giant brand American
Mixtures, Manhattan Style" (Broccoli, cauliflower, pea
pods, and red peppers.)
3 - Chicken breast halves, boneless and skinned.
1/4 - Cup canola oil
2 - Tablespoons sesame seed oil
2 - Eggs, lightly beaten
1/2 - Teaspoon salt
Soy sauce (to taste when served)

Instructions:

Thaw vegetables to room temperature and heat 4
tablespoons canola oil mixed with 1 tablespoon sesame
oil on medium in a wok. Remove any excess fat from
chicken and cut chicken into bite size pieces. Cook
chicken in the canola and olive oil until done. Remove
cooked chicken and discard the oil and juices in wok.
Heat 2 tablespoons canola oil mixed with 1 tablespoon
sesame oil on medium heat in the wok. Add the
packages of thawed vegetables and stir fry until tender.
Add additional oil if needed to prevent the vegetables
from browning. In a small bowl, beat eggs with a fork.
Slowly pour the beaten eggs into the vegetables and
continue stir frying until the eggs are cooked and in small
bits. Add the cooked chicken and continue to stir fry until
the chicken is heated. Sprinkle with soy sauce to taste
and serve.
Serves 3

Category of Recipe: Poultry

Name of Recipe: Grilled Sesame Chicken

Recipe Color Code: Red

Ingredients:

6 - Chicken breast halves, skinless and boneless
1/4 - Cup melted butter or margarine
1/4 - Cup sesame seeds (see note in instructions below)
2 - Teaspoons lemon juice
1 - Teaspoon dried basil
1 - Teaspoon salt
1/2 - Teaspoon ground black pepper

Instructions:

Cut 6 pieces of aluminum foil, each piece being large enough to hold one of the chicken breast halves and still have approximately 1 inch of foil to turn up on the edges to prevent the juices from running out while grilling - do not punch holes in the foil. Combine other ingredients, except the basil, and mix well. Using about half of the sauce, generously brush the mixture on one side of each piece of chicken and place the brushed side down on the aluminum foil. Grill about 4 or 5 inches from heat for 5 to 8 minutes (or until about half done). Baste with remaining sauce, turn, sprinkle cooked side with basil, and cook for 5 additional minutes or until done. Serve on the foil.
Serves 4 to 6

Note: Sesame seeds may be first browned by mixing with 1 teaspoon of melted butter/margarine and micro waving on high for 5 minutes, stirring every 2 minutes minimum.

Category of Recipe: | Poultry

Name of Recipe: | Chicken Salad with Pecans on Lettuce

Recipe Color Code: | Red

Ingredients:

6 - Chicken breast halves, boneless and skinless
2 - Teaspoons white pepper
1 - Cup celery, finely chopped
1/2 - Cup scallions, finely chopped
1/4 - Cup shallots, finely chopped
3/4 - Cup canola oil mayonnaise
1/4 - Cup Dijon mustard
1/4 - Cup fresh parsley, chopped
1/2 - Pecans, chopped
1 - Head iceberg lettuce, shredded

Instructions:

Pre-heat broiler. Season the chicken breast halves with 1 teaspoon white pepper, then broil until fully cooked, about 6 minutes per side. Refrigerate the cooked chicken until cold, then chop them into a large dice. Place the diced chicken in a large bowl and combine with the celery, scallions, shallots, mayonnaise, mustard, remaining white pepper, and parsley. Mix well and chill completely before serving. Spread the pecans on a pie pan and toast about 5 minutes in an oven preheated to 300 degrees. Let cool. Arrange a bed of shredded lettuce on 6 chilled serving plates. For each serving, pack salad into a 1 cup mold, then invert onto the lettuce beds. Sprinkle each salad with toasted pecans and serve.
Serves 6 to 8

Category of Recipe: | Poultry

Name of Recipe: | Deviled Eggs

Recipe Color Code: | Red

Ingredients:

6 - Large eggs
1 - Teaspoon prepared mustard
1 - Teaspoon Dijon mustard
1/2 - Teaspoon salt
1 - Tablespoon fresh chives, chopped
1/2 - Teaspoon ground black pepper
3 - Tablespoons canola oil mayonnaise
Paprika for garnish

Instructions:

Place the eggs in a pan and cover them with cold tap water. Place the pan on medium-high heat and bring to a boil. Reduce the heat to a simmer and cook for 15 minutes. Rinse the eggs under cold water and peel. Allow the eggs to cool in a refrigerator for 15 minutes. Halve the eggs lengthwise and carefully scoop out the yolks. In a bowl, mash the yolks with a fork and add the mustard, salt, pepper, and chives. Fold in the mayonnaise. Fill the whites with the egg yolk mixture and sprinkle the tops with paprika.
Serves 4 to 6

Category of Recipe: Poultry

Name of Recipe: Chicken with Caramelized Onion Sauce

Recipe Color Code: Red

Ingredients:

4 - Chicken breast halves, skinless and boneless
1 - Tablespoon olive oil
1 - Large onion, thinly sliced
2 - Cups water
Salt to taste
Ground black pepper to taste

Instructions:

In a large skillet, heat the olive oil on medium and add the chicken. Brown both sides of each piece. Reduce heat and sauté chicken for approximately 10 minutes. Add salt and pepper to taste. Add the sliced onion to the skillet and stir together with the chicken for approximately 5 minutes. Add 2 cups of water and let simmer on medium heat until the onion caramelizes and creates a sauce. Simmer for approximately 30 minutes. You might need to add more water so that the sauce mixture doesn't dry out. Once the chicken is cooked thoroughly, remove and place each piece on a serving plate. Top with the caramelized onion sauce and serve.
Serves 4

Category of Recipe: Poultry

Name of Recipe: Chicken Parmigiania

Recipe Color Code: Red

Ingredients:

8 - Chicken breast halves, skinless and boneless
3 - Tablespoons olive oil
1 - Large onion, finely chopped (approximately 1 cup)
1 - Clove garlic, crushed
1 - 28 ounce can peeled and dices tomatoes, drained
1 - 14 ounce can peeled and diced tomatoes, drained
1 - Teaspoon salt
1/2 - Teaspoon freshly ground black pepper
1 - Teaspoon leaf basil, crumbled
1 - Teaspoon leaf oregano, crumbled
1/2 - Teaspoon nutmeg
1/2 - Cup canola oil
1 1/2 - Cups (6-8 ounces) shredded Mozzarella cheese
1/2 - Cup (2 ounces) grated Parmesan cheese
2 - Eggs, lightly beaten

Instructions:

Pre-heat oven to 350 degrees. Heat olive oil in a medium saucepan. Place the chopped onion in the olive oil and sauté until tender but not browned. Add the garlic and cook 1 minute. Add tomatoes and cook on medium heat uncovered, for 15 minutes to thicken. Add basil, oregano, salt, pepper, nutmeg and stir. Cook over medium heat an additional 10 minutes, stirring often. In a large heavy skillet, heat 1/4 cup canola oil on medium. Place chicken between sheets of wax paper and pound with meat mallet until the chicken is about 1/4 inch thick. Dip chicken in the beaten eggs. Cook chicken in the canola oil, 1 layer at a time, until done and slightly brown on both sides. Add canola oil as need for frying. Spray an 8" x 10" baking dish with a non-stick cooking spray, cover the bottom with 4 tablespoons of the cooked tomato sauce, and alternate (2) layers as follows: Chicken, tomato sauce, Mozzarella cheese, Parmesan cheese (ending with the Mozzarella cheese topped with Parmesan. Bake at 350 degrees for 22 minutes or until cheese has melted and the dish is bubbly hot. Let set for 1- to 15 minutes before serving. Divide into 6 servings.

Category of Recipe: | Poultry

Name of Recipe: | Baked Chicken Breast with Tarragon

Recipe Color Code: | Red

Ingredients:

1 - Cup low fat buttermilk
2 - Green onions (or one medium white) chopped.
2 - Teaspoons paprika
1 - Level teaspoon dried tarragon (measure accurately)
1 - Teaspoon garlic powder
1/2 - Teaspoon freshly ground black pepper
4 - Chicken breast halves, boneless and skinless

Instructions:

Pre-heat oven to 325 degrees. Combine all the ingredients, except the chicken, in a bowl and mix until blended. Spray a 13 inch x 9 inch baking dish with non-stick spray. Place the chicken in the baking dish, and then pour half of the mixture over the chicken. Turn the chicken several times to coat, and then pour the other half of the mixture over the chicken. Bake at 325 degrees for 45 minutes, turning chicken twice (about every 15 minutes) until cooked thoroughly.
Serves 4

Category of Recipe: Poultry

Name of Recipe: French Baked Chicken

Recipe Color Code: Red

Ingredients:

2 - Chicken breast halves, boneless and skinless
1 - Cup onion, thinly sliced
2 - Cloves garlic, minced
2 - Cups mushrooms, sliced
2 - Medium tomatoes, cored and cut into 4 pieces each
1/3 - Cup white wine, dry preferred
2 - Tablespoons vinegar
1 - Teaspoon dried thyme, crumbled
1/2 - Teaspoon salt
1/2 - Teaspoon ground black pepper

Instructions:

Spray a large non-stick skillet with non-stick cooking spray; add the chicken breasts and cook over medium heat, turning occasionally, until the chicken is browned on both sides (about 10 to 12 minutes). Spray a 13 inch by 9 inch baking dish with non-stick cooking spray; transfer the browned chicken to the baking dish and set aside. Pre-heat oven to 350 degrees. Place onion and garlic in same skillet in which the chicken was browned, and cook over medium-low heat, stirring occasionally, until the onion is tender (about 10 minutes). Add mushrooms, and stir. Cook 3 minutes longer. Stir in remaining ingredients and cook an additional 2 minutes, stirring often. Pour the vegetable mixture evenly over the chicken. Cover the baking dish with aluminum foi8l and bake 25 minutes. Remove foil and bake an additional 20 minutes uncovered.
Serves 4

Category of Recipe: | Poultry

Name of Recipe: | Turkey Divan

Recipe Color Code: | Red

Ingredients:

1 1/2 - Pounds fresh broccoli (or 2 - 10 ounce frozen).
1/2 - Teaspoon dried whole oregano
1/2 - Teaspoon salt
1/2 - Cup sugar-free mayonnaise
1/4 - Cup (1 ounce) shredded cheddar cheese
2 - Tablespoons grated Parmesan cheese
1/4 - Cup low fat milk
8 to 12 - Slices cooked turkey breast

Instructions:

Trim off large leaves of broccoli and remove tough ends;
wash thoroughly and cut into spears. Place broccoli in a
shallow 2 - quart baking dish, with stem ends toward
outside of dish; add oregano and 1/2 cup water. Cover
with lid or heavy-duty plastic wrap, and microwave on
high for 8 minutes, stir, and cook an additional 3 minutes
on high power; or, until broccoli is tender. Drain and
place in 4 individual serving dishes. Sprinkle with salt.
Place approximately 3 ounces sliced turkey on each
serving of broccoli (may be 2 or 3 loose rolled slices on
each). Combine the mayonnaise, cheddar cheese, and
milk in a 2 cup glass measuring cup. Microwave on
medium high (70% power) for 1 to 2 minutes or until
cheese melts, stirring after 1 minute. Stir again and
spoon 1/4 of the mixture over each of the four servings.
Sprinkle Parmesan cheese over sauce as desired.
Serves 4

Category of Recipe: Poultry

Name of Recipe: Baked Spicy Chicken

Recipe Color Code: Red

Ingredients:
1 - Tablespoon tomato ketchup
1 - Tablespoon red wine vinegar
2 - Teaspoons canola oil
2 - Cloves garlic, minced
2 - Teaspoons ginger root, minced
1/2 - Teaspoon ground red pepper (optional)
1/4 - Teaspoon ground cinnamon
1/8 - Teaspoon freshly ground black pepper
4 - Chicken breast halves, boneless and skinless

Instructions:
Pre-heat oven to 325 degrees. Combine all ingredients, except the chicken, in a small bowl. Place chicken in an 11 inch by 7 inch baking dish; brush both sides of the chicken pieces with the mixture. Bake for 45 minutes, or until tender and cooked through; turn once after 25 minutes.
Serves 4

Category of Recipe: Salads and Dressings

Name of Recipe: Mexican Layer Dip

Recipe Color Code: Red

Ingredients:

1 - 16 ounce can refried beans
chili powder
1 - 8 ounce container sour cream
1 - 8 ounce jar plicate sauce of choice
6 - Ounces guacamole
3 - Tomatoes, diced
1 - 8 ounce jar sliced jalapeno peppers
8 - Ounces finely grated sharp cheddar cheese
1 - 8 ounce jar black olives, sliced

Instructions:

On a large platter or shallow dish, lay refried beans, sprinkle chili powder, add sour cream and the remainder of ingredients in the order given.
Serves 8 to 10

Category of Recipe: Salads and Dressings

Name of Recipe: Onion Dressing

Recipe Color Code: Yellow

Ingredients:

1/2 - Large onion; Vidalia preferred
2 - Cups canola oil mayonnaise
1 - Teaspoon Dijon mustard
1 - Teaspoon paprika
2 - Packages artificial sweetener
1/2 - Teaspoon ground black pepper
1/2 - Teaspoon turmeric
1/4 - Teaspoon garlic powder
1/4 - Cup white vinegar

Instructions:

Place onion in food processor and process until finely chopped. Mix remaining ingredients in processor with the onion and process until well blended. Keep refrigerated.
Serves 8 to 12

Category of Recipe:	Salads and Dressings
Name of Recipe:	Blue Cheese Salad Dressing (or Dip)
Recipe Color Code:	Red

Ingredients:

4 - Ounces blue cheese, crumbled
1/2- Teaspoon garlic, crushed
2 - Cups canola oil mayonnaise
1 - Cup sour cream
1/4 - Cup white wine vinegar
1 - Teaspoon lemon juice
1/4 - Teaspoon ground black pepper
1/2 - Teaspoon fresh parsley, finely chopped
1/2 - Teaspoon salt

Instructions:

Crumble the cheese into a large mixing bowl. Remove 1/2 the crumbled cheese and set aside. Add other ingredients into the mixing bowl and blend together until all the cheese lumps are smooth. This may be done by using a mixer or a food processor. Using a spatula, stir in the remaining crumbled cheese until evenly distributed throughout (do not blend the second half of blue cheese). Keep refrigerated in a glass or plastic container.
Serves 8 to 12

Category of Recipe: | Salads and Dressings

Name of Recipe: | Seven Layer Salad

Recipe Color Code: | Red

Ingredients:

1 - Cup chopped celery
3 - Cups head lettuce, chopped into bite size pieces
4 - Hard boiled eggs, chopped
1/4 - Cup chopped onion
1/4 - Cup chopped green bell pepper
1 - Cup frozen peas
1 1/2 - Cups canola oil mayonnaise
1 - Packet artificial sweetener
1/3 - Cup shredded cheddar cheese
1/4 - Cup cooked bacon, chopped

Instructions:

Using a 1 1/2 quart casserole dish, layer items 1 through 6 in the order listed above. In a separate bowl, mix mayonnaise with the artificial sweetener and mix well. Spread the mayonnaise mixture evenly over the last item (peas) in the casserole dish. Top the mayonnaise mixture by evenly sprinkling with the shredded cheese and chopped cooked bacon.
Serves 6 to 8

Note: Better if allowed sitting in the refrigerator for a minim of 4 hours, preferably overnight, before serving.

Category of Recipe: Salads and Dressings

Name of Recipe: Dijon Vinaigrette Salad Dressing

Recipe Color Code: Yellow

Ingredients:

1/4 - Cup Grey Poupon mustard
1 1/4 - Cups canola or olive oil
1/2 - Cup red wine vinegar

Instructions:

Thoroughly mix all ingredients and serve.
Serves 8

Category of Recipe: | Salads and Dressings

Name of Recipe: | Chef Salad

Recipe Color Code: | Red

Ingredients:

1 – cup shredded lettuce
1 – hard-boiled egg, sliced
2 – ounces cooked turkey or chicken breast, sliced
2 – ounces cooked ham, sliced
¼ - cup cucumber, sliced
6 – cherry tomatoes
½ - cup salad dressing of choice

Instructions:

In a large bowl, add all ingredients. Toss with dressing.
Serve immediately.
Serves 2

Category of Recipe: | Salads and Dressings

Name of Recipe: | Cobb Salad

Recipe Color Code: | Red

Ingredients:

2 - Cups (about 10 ounces) cooked turkey breast, cut
    into bite size pieces
9 - Slices crisp cooked bacon, bite size pieces
4 - Eggs, hard boiled and chopped
5 - Cups chopped iceberg lettuce
2 - Tomatoes, diced into bite size pieces
3/4 - Cup bleu cheese, crumbled
1 - Medium avocado, diced into about 1/2 inch pieces
Salt and pepper to taste
Salad dressing as follows (or other of choice):
   1/3 - Cup olive oil
   2 - Tablespoons red wine vinegar
   2 - Teaspoons Dijon mustard
   2 - Garlic cloves, minced
   Salt and ground black pepper to taste

Instructions:

On serving plates, form mounds of chopped lettuce. The
other salad ingredients, except those in the dressing,
may either be layered individually on the lettuce or they
may be placed in individual pie shaped sections on top of
the lettuce. Mix the dressing ingredients and serve on
the side.
Serves 4

Category of Recipe: Salads and Dressings

Name of Recipe: Pea Salad

Recipe Color Code: Red

Ingredients:

1 – 15 ounce can early small peas, drained
1 – cup cubed Cheddar cheese (about ¼ inch cubes)
½ - cup chopped celery
½ - cup sliced pimento-stuffed olives
1 – hard-boiled egg, chopped
1 – tablespoon finely chopped onion
¼ - cup mayonnaise

Instructions:

Combine all ingredients and mix well. Cover salad and chill for at least 1 hour.
Serves 4

Category of Recipe: Salads and Dressings

Name of Recipe: Sweet and Sour Dressing

Recipe Color Code: Yellow

Ingredients:

1 - Cup vegetable oil
1/2 - Cup vinegar
8 - Packages artificial sweetener of choice
1 - Teaspoon salt
1 - Teaspoon celery seeds
1 - Teaspoon paprika
1 - Teaspoon grated onion

Instructions:

Combine all ingredients in a jar. Cover tightly and shake vigorously. Chill several hours. Shade again before serving over salad. Yield is 1 3/4 cups.
Serves 4

Category of Recipe: | Salads and Dressings

Name of Recipe: | Italian Vinaigrette Dressing

Recipe Color Code: | Yellow

Ingredients:

3/4 - Cup olive oil
1/3 - Cup red wine vinegar
2 - Teaspoons Dijon mustard
1/8 - Teaspoon salt
1/8 - Teaspoon ground black pepper
1 - Teaspoon grated Parmesan cheese (optional)

Instructions:

Place all the ingredients, except the cheese, in a small bowl. Hold a wire whisk upright in the bowl and rotate it between the palms of your hands until the vinaigrette is well blended. For an Italian accent, add Parmesan cheese and mix.
Serves 8 to 10

Category of Recipe:	Salads and Dressings
Name of Recipe:	Cucumber Mint Salad
Recipe Color Code:	Yellow

Ingredients:

2 - Large cucumbers
1/2 - Teaspoon coarse (kosher) salt
1 - Cup plain low-fat yogurt
1 - Tablespoon olive oil
2 - Teaspoons white wine vinegar
2 - Packages artificial sweetener
1 - Teaspoon salt
1/2 - Teaspoon ground black pepper
2 - Tablespoons chopped fresh mint leaves
4 - Radishes, very thinly sliced, for garnish
Mint sprigs for garnish

Instructions:

Peel the cucumbers, cut then in half lengthwise, and remove the seeds. Slice the halves into thin crescents. Lay them on paper towels, sprinkle with the coarse salt, and refrigerate, uncovered, for 1 hour. Remove the cucumbers from the refrigerator and pat dry. Combine the yogurt, oil, vinegar, sweetener, salt, pepper, and mint in a small bowl. Blend thoroughly, and toss with the cucumbers. Divide equally onto salad plates and decorate with the radishes and min sprigs, serve immediately.
Serves 2 to 4

Category of Recipe: Salads and Dressings

Name of Recipe: Salad with Feta and Olives

Recipe Color Code: Red

Ingredients:

1 - Medium red onion, thinly slice and separate into rings
2 - Tablespoons red wine vinegar (for onion)
1 - Heart of romaine lettuce, shredded
3 - Large tomatoes, peeled and chopped
1 - Cucumber, peeled, seeded, and chopped
1 - Green bell pepper, seeded and diced
1 - Bunch radishes, sliced
1/2 - Cup oil-cured black olives
2 - Cups (8 ounces) crumbled feta cheese
Following items for the dressing:
　1/2 - Cup red wine vinegar
　2 - Tablespoons lemon juice
　1/2 - Teaspoon oregano
　1 - Package artificial sweetener of choice
　1/2 - Cup olive oil
　½ teaspoon salt and ¼ teaspoon ground black pepper

Instructions:

Place the onion rings and vinegar in a large bowl. Sprinkle with 1 teaspoon salt, toss to coat, and using your hands, work the onion, vinegar, and salt together for several minutes. Let stand 20 minutes. Add the romaine, tomatoes, cucumber, green pepper, celery, radishes, olives, and feta to the onion rings. Toss to mix. In a small bowl or screw top jar, beat together or shake the vinegar, lemon juice, sweetener, oil, ½ teaspoon salt, and ¼ teaspoon ground black pepper. Pour over the salad and toss. Serve immediately.
Serves 6 to 8

Category of Recipe: Salads and Dressings

Name of Recipe: Sugar Free Cole Slaw

Recipe Color Code: Yellow

Ingredients:

1 - Large or 2 small heads cabbage, shredded
2 - Medium onions, chopped
1 - Medium green bell pepper, chopped
3 - Cups canola oil mayonnaise
2 - Tablespoons Dijon mustard
1 - Tablespoon celery seed
6 - Tablespoon lemon juice
4 - Packages artificial sweetener of choice
Salt to taste
Pepper to taste

Instructions:

Combine mayonnaise, mustard, celery seed, lemon juice
and sweetener. Mix well. To prepare slaw, toss
cabbage, peppers and onions together. Toss dressing
with slaw, salt and pepper. Refrigerate before serving.
Serves 6

Category of Recipe: | Salads and Dressings

Name of Recipe: | Quick Tuna Salad

Recipe Color Code: | Red

Ingredients:

2 - 6 ounce cans tuna fish, drained
2 - Tablespoons canola oil mayonnaise
3 - Tablespoons chopped pickles or relish of choice

Instructions:

Mix all ingredients well. Keep refrigerated if not served immediately.
Serves 4

Category of Recipe: Salads and Dressings

Name of Recipe: Green Goddess Salad Dressing

Recipe Color Code: Red

Ingredients:

9 or 10 - Anchovy filets
1 - Green onion
1/4 - Cup fresh parsley, minced
2 - Tablespoons fresh tarragon, minced
3 - Cups canola oil mayonnaise
1/4 - Cup tarragon vinegar
1/2 - Cup chives, minced

Instructions:

Mince the green onion with the anchovy. Add the parsley, tarragon, mayonnaise, vinegar and chives. Mix well. Refrigerate in a tightly covered container until serving.
Serves 8 to 10

Category of Recipe: | Salads and Dressings

Name of Recipe: | Caesar Salad

Recipe Color Code: | Red

Ingredients:

1 – large head romaine lettuce
2/3 – cup olive oil
3 – tablespoons red wine vinegar
1 – tablespoon Worcestershire sauce
½ - teaspoon Dijon mustard
½ - teaspoon salt
1 – clove garlic, crushed
1 – lemon, halved
Freshly ground black pepper to taste
¼ - cup grated Parmesan cheese

Instructions:

Wash lettuce under cold running water. Trim core and separate lettuce into leaves. Discard wilted or discolored portions. Shake leaves well to remove moisture. Place in a large plastic bag and chill at least 2 hours. Combine olive oil, vinegar, Worcestershire sauce, salt, mustard, and garlic in a jar. Tightly cover, shake vigorously and set aside. Cut course ribs from large leaves of lettuce. Tear leaves into bite size pieces and place on a large salad bowl. Pour dressing over the lettuce. Toss gently until the lettuce is well coated. Squeeze juice from lemon halves over salad. Grind a generous amount of black pepper over the salad, sprinkle with cheese and toss. Top with cooked and sliced chicken breast and/or crisp bacon if desired. Serve immediately.
Serves 4 to 6

Category of Recipe:	Salads and Dressings

Name of Recipe:	Broccoli Salad

Recipe Color Code:	Yellow

Ingredients:

¾ - cup canola oil or light mayonnaise
½ - cup sour cream
6 – packets artificial sweetener of choice
3 – tablespoons French dressing (do not use low-fat)
2- tablespoons Balsamic vinegar (optional)
2 – heads broccoli, broken into bite size pieces
5 – slices cooked bacon, crumbled
1/2 – medium red onion, sliced
2 – cups cherry salad tomatoes, cut in half

Instructions:

Combine and mix all ingredients.
Serves 4 to 6

Note: Refrigerate left over salad; just as good the second day.

Category of Recipe: | Salads and Dressings

Name of Recipe: | Buttermilk Ranch Salad Dressing

Recipe Color Code: | Red

Ingredients:

3 – cloves garlic, finely minced
¾ - canola oil
½ - cup fresh lemon juice (about 4 lemons)
½ - cup canola or light mayonnaise
1/3 – cup buttermilk
1 ½ - teaspoon dill weed, dried
1 – packet artificial sweetener
1 ½ - teaspoon coarsely ground black pepper
1 – teaspoon salt

Instructions:

Process the garlic in a food processor until finely minced. Add the remaining ingredients and process until smooth and thickened.

Category of Recipe: | Salads and Dressings

Name of Recipe: | Home Style Mayonnaise (sugar free)

Recipe Color Code: | Yellow

Ingredients:

1 – whole large egg
1 – teaspoon Dijon mustard
1 – teaspoon lemon juice
1 – tablespoon canola oil
¼ - teaspoon salt
1 – packet artificial sweetener
1 – cup canola oil

Instructions:

Process the first 6 ingredients in a food processor on high speed for about 4 or 5 seconds. With processor running on high speed, very slowly pour the cup of canola oil into the mixture (use the processor feeder tube with the small hole). The mixture should begin to thicken almost immediately. Spoon the mayonnaise into a glass or plastic container, cover and chill. (Do not store in a metal container.)
Number of servings depends on use.

Category of Recipe: | Sauces

Name of Recipe: | Tartar Sauce

Recipe Color Code: | Yellow

Ingredients:

1 - Cup canola oil mayonnaise
1 - Tablespoon fresh lemon juice
1 - Teaspoon lemon zest, finely grated
1 - Teaspoon tomato paste
1 - Teaspoon Dijon mustard
2 - Tablespoons dill pickle, very finely chopped
2 - Tablespoons shallots, finely chopped
2 - Tablespoons fresh parsley, finely chopped
1 - Teaspoon jalapeno pepper, finely chopped (optional)
1 - Tablespoon capers, drained
Salt and pepper to taste

Instructions:

In a bowl, combine the mayonnaise, mustard, tomato paste, lemon juice, lemon zest, and pickles. Mix in parsley jalapeno pepper, shallots and capers. Salt and pepper to taste and refrigerate for at least 1 hour before serving.
Serves 6 to 8

Category of Recipe: | Sauces

Name of Recipe: | Fresh Southwestern Salsa

Recipe Color Code: | Yellow

Ingredients:

10 - Medium tomatoes, quartered
1/2 - Cup chopped onion
1/2 - Cup chopped green onion with stems
1 - Large jalapeno pepper, quartered, seeded (optional)
2 - Tablespoons chopped fresh cilantro
1 1/2 - Packages artificial sweetener
1 - Teaspoon ground black pepper
1 - Teaspoon lime juice
1 1/2 - Teaspoons salt

Instructions:

In a food processor, combine tomatoes, onion, green onions, jalapeno pepper, and cilantro. Process until sauce is just chunky. Pour into large mixing bowl. Stir in sweetener, black pepper, lime juice, and salt. Cover and store in refrigerator for up to two weeks. Serve as an appetizer dip or a sauce for fish, chicken, beef, or pork. Serves 12

Category of Recipe: | Sauces

Name of Recipe: | Marinara Sauce

Recipe Color Code: | Yellow

Ingredients:

1 - 28 ounce can Italian tomatoes
1 - 6 ounce can tomato sauce
4 - Tablespoons fresh parsley, chopped
1 - Garlic clove, minced
1 - Teaspoons dried oregano
1 - Teaspoon salt
1/4 - Teaspoon ground black pepper
6 - Tablespoon olive oil
1/3 - Cup finely chopped onion
1/2 - Cup dry white wine

Instructions:

Place Italian tomatoes, tomato paste, chopped parsley, minced garlic, oregano, salt, and pepper in a food processor; process until smooth. In a large skillet over medium heat, sauté the chopped onion in olive oil for 2 minutes. Add the blended tomato sauce and wine. Simmer for approximately 30 minutes, stirring frequently to prevent scorching.
Serves 6 to 8

Category of Recipe:	Sauces

Name of Recipe:	Tomato Ketchup (sugar free)

Recipe Color Code:	Yellow

Ingredients:

1 - 6 ounce can Contadina brand tomato paste
1 - 15 ounce can Contadina brand tomato sauce
2 - Tablespoons red wine vinegar
1 1/2 - Teaspoons onion powder
1/4 - Teaspoon salt
2 - Packages artificial sweetener

Instructions:

Place all ingredients, except sweetener, in a sauce pan and mix thoroughly. Simmer on low heat for approximately 10 minutes, stirring frequently to prevent scorching. Set aside and let cool to room temperature. Add the sweetener and mix thoroughly.
Serves 12 to 15

Category of Recipe: | Seafood

Name of Recipe: | Fried Salmon with Herbs, Sherry and Almonds

Recipe Color Code: | Red

Ingredients:

1/4 - Teaspoon onion salt
1/4 - Teaspoon dried oregano
1/4 - Teaspoon dried parsley
1/2 - Teaspoon dried tarragon
1/4 - Teaspoon ground black pepper
1 - Small clove garlic, minced
1/4 - Cup plus 2 tablespoons butter or margarine, melted
2 1/4 - Pounds (2 filets) fresh salmon (or favorite fish)
1 cup thinly sliced almonds
3 tablespoons cooking sherry
1 bunch fresh parsley for garnish (optional)

Instructions:

Sauté seasonings and garlic in butter in a large heavy skillet over medium heat for 1 minute. Reduce heat to medium-low; add fish (skin side up). Cook fish, covered, for eight minutes. Turn and cook an additional 8 minutes, covered, or until fish flakes easily when tested with a fork (do no overcook). Remove fish with a slotted turner, place on a heated platter with skin side down, and keep warm. Put almonds in same skillet and brown for 2 to 3 minutes, stirring frequently. Pour sherry into skillet with toasted almonds, stir, and cook over high heat for 30 to 45 seconds. Pour sherry and almond mixture evenly over fish, garnish with parsley, and serve immediately. Serves 4

Notes: Cooking times vary depending on size, thickness, and kind of filet. Simply cook until done and slightly browned. This is an absolutely delicious dish!

Category of Recipe: | Seafood

Name of Recipe: | Crab Cakes

Recipe Color Code: | Red

Ingredients:

1 – pound crab meat, free of shells and cartilage
1 – egg, lightly beaten
1 – tablespoon Dijon mustard
½ - teaspoon Worcestershire sauce
2 ½ - teaspoons lemon juice
½ - teaspoon Old Bay Seasoning
1 - whole green onion, chopped
½ - green sweet bell pepper, finely chopped
¼ - cup buttermilk
¾ - cup bread crumbs, made from processing 1 slice
     of *Ezekiel 4:9* bread (sugar free and flour free)
½ - teaspoon salt
¼ - teaspoon ground black pepper
4 – tablespoons canola oil
2 – tablespoons butter

Instructions:

Process the slice of bread into crumbs, using a food processor. Lightly beat the egg. Heat 2 tablespoon of the canola oil in a heavy skillet over medium heat. Sauté the onion and bell pepper until tender (about 3 minutes after the oil is heated). Place the sautéed onion and pepper in a large mixing bowl. Add the egg, mustard, Worcestershire sauce, lemon juice, Old Bay seasoning, buttermilk, breadcrumbs, salt, and black pepper. Gently mix all the ingredients and then fold in the crab meat. Add the other 2 tablespoons of canola oil and the 2 tablespoons butter to the heavy skillet and re-heat over medium heat. Form the crab meat mixture into 8 patties of about ½ inch thick each. Cook the patties in the oil and butter mixture until golden brown, about 3 minutes. Gently turn the patties and cook on the other side for about 3 minutes until also golden brown. Note: depending on the size of the skillet, it might be that only 4 can be cooked at a time. Serve with a side of mustard, vinegar or sauce of choice for dipping.
Serves 6 to 8

Category of Recipe: Seafood

Name of Recipe: Shrimp Creole

Recipe Color Code: Red

Ingredients:

1 1/2 - Pounds unpeeled fresh shrimp
1 - Medium onion, chopped
1 - Medium green bell pepper, chopped
1 - Cup celery, chopped
1 - Cup okra, sliced
2 - Cloves garlic, minced
3 - Tablespoons canola oil
1 - 16 ounce can diced tomatoes, un-drained
1 - 8 ounce can tomato sauce
2 - Teaspoons Worcestershire sauce
1/2 - Teaspoon dried oregano
1/2 - Teaspoon dried thyme
1/4 - Teaspoons nutmeg
1/2 - Teaspoon salt
1 - Teaspoon Cajun seasoning of choice
1 - Cup converted rice

Instructions:

Steam shrimp for approximately 3 minutes (9 minutes for frozen shrimp), or until shrimp turns pink in color; immediately dump the cooked shrimp into a colander to drain, then run cold tap water over them to stop them from cooking any more. Peal, de-vein, and set cooked shrimp aside. In a large deep skillet, heat the canola oil over medium-low heat and sauté onion, green pepper, celery, okra, and garlic until tender. Stir in tomatoes, tomato sauce, Worcestershire sauce, oregano, thyme, salt, nutmeg, and Cajun seasoning. Cook over medium heat, stirring occasionally, about 15 minutes or until desired consistency. Stir in shrimp, and simmer over medium heat approximately 2 minutes or until shrimp are reheated. Serve over rice.

Serves 4 to 6

Note: To cook rice, add 2 chicken or beef bouillon cubes to 2 1/2 cups water. Bring to boil, add 1 cup rice, bring back to boil and turn heat down to medium-low heat. Cover and cook 1 hour. Do not remove lid during the hour of cooking or the grains of rice will stick together.

Category of Recipe: Seafood

Name of Recipe: Tarragon Fish

Recipe Color Code: Red

Ingredients:

2 - Orange roughly fish filets (about 1/2 pound each)
2 - Tablespoons olive oil
2 - Tablespoons tarragon
2 - Cloves garlic, crushed

Instructions:

Rinse and drain fish. Place olive oil in skillet and heat on medium heat. Add tarragon; heat and stir just until warm. Spread mixture evenly over skillet. Add fish and cover. Cook over medium heat for about 10 minutes on each side, or until fish flakes with fork.
Serves 2 to 3

Category of Recipe: | Seafood

Name of Recipe: | Shrimp Scampi

Recipe Color Code: | Red

Ingredients:

2 - Pounds medium size, fresh shrimp
1/4 - Cup green onions with stems, chopped
1/4 - Cup fresh parsley, chopped
3 - Cloves garlic, crushed
3/4 - Cup butter or margarine, melted
1/4 - Cup dry white wine
2 - Tablespoons lemon juice
3/4 - Teaspoon salt
1/4 - Teaspoon ground black pepper

Instructions:

Pour water into bottom a steamer, about 3/4 inch deep. Bring water to boil and steam shrimp, covered, for approximately 3 minutes or until they turn pink in color. Immediately dump shrimp into a colander to drain, then run cold tap water over them to stop them from cooking any more. Peel, De-vein, and set cooked shrimp aside. (If shrimp are frozen, cook for a total of 9 minutes.) In a skillet, melt the butter over medium-low heat. Sauté green onions, parsley, and garlic until onions are tender. Reduce heat to low and add the cooked shrimp while continuously stirring, again heating for approximately 1 minute. Remove only the shrimp, with a slotted spoon, to four individual serving dishes. Add remaining ingredients to the butter mixture. Stir and simmer for 2 additional minutes. Pour butter mixture equally over each dish of shrimp.
Serves 3 to 4

Category of Recipe:	Seafood
Name of Recipe:	Crock Pot Shrimp Creole
Recipe Color Code:	Red

Ingredients:

1 1/2 - Cups onion, chopped
3/4 - Cup celery, chopped
1 - Garlic clove, minced
3/4 - Cup green bell pepper, diced
1 - 28 ounce can whole tomatoes
2 - 8 ounce cans tomato sauce
1/2 - Teaspoon salt
1/4 - Teaspoon ground black pepper
1 - Teaspoon paprika
1 - Bay leaf
1/4 - Teaspoon hot sauce of choice
1 - Pound fresh shrimp, shelled and de-veined (or 1 - 16
     ounce package frozen shelled shrimp, rinsed
     and drained)

Instructions:

Combine all ingredients, except shrimp, in crock pot; stir well to blend. Cover; cook on high for 3 hours. Add shrimp and cook on high for 1 additional hour, or until the shrimp turn pink. (Additional hot sauce may be added to taste.)
Serves 6

Category of Recipe: | Seafood

Name of Recipe: | Creole Jambalaya

Recipe Color Code: | Red

Ingredients:

1/2 - Cup olive oil
3 - Cups onion, chopped
2 - Tablespoons minced shallots
2 - Cloves garlic, minced
2 - Medium green bell peppers, chopped
3 - Teaspoons salt
1 - Pound smoked sausage, cut into bite size pieces
3 - Chicken breast halves, skinless and boneless, cut
    into bite size pieces
1 - Teaspoon cayenne pepper
2 - Teaspoons hot sauce
3 - Bay leaves
3 - Cups converted rice
6 - Cups water
1 - Cup green onions, chopped

Instructions:

Heat the oil in a large heavy pot. Add the onions, shallots, garlic, bell pepper, 2 teaspoons of the salt and cayenne pepper. Stir and brown the vegetables for about 20 minutes, or until they reach a dark caramelized color. Add the sausage and continue the browning procedure, stirring often and scraping the bottom and sides of the pot to loosen any browned particles, cooking for about 15 minutes. Season the chicken with the remaining salt. Add chicken to the pot, along with the bay leaves. Add the rice and stir for 3 minutes. Add the hot sauce and water. Stir and cover. Cook for 35 minutes, or until the rice is tender and the liquid has been absorbed. Remove from heat and let stand 3 minutes. Garnish with green onions.
Serves 8 to 10

Category of Recipe: | Seafood

Name of Recipe: | Grilled Sesame Fish

Recipe Color Code: | Red

Ingredients:

6 - Fish filets of choice
1/4 - Cup melted butter or margarine
1/4 - Cup sesame seeds
2 - Teaspoons lemon juice
1 - Teaspoon salt
1/2 - Teaspoon ground black pepper

Instructions:

Cut 6 pieces of aluminum foil, large enough to hold a fish filet and still have approximately 1 inch of foil to turn up on the edges to prevent the juices from running out - do not punch holes in the foil. Combine other ingredients and mix well. Brush mixture on one side of fish (opposite the side which has any skin) and place the brushed side down on the aluminum foil. Cook about 4 inches from heat for 5 to 8 minutes (slightly longer if the filets are thick). Baste with remaining sauce, turn, and cook 5 additional minutes or until fish flakes easily with a fork. Serve on the foil.
Serves 6

Category of Recipe: | Seafood

Name of Recipe: | Spicy Broiled Fish Filets

Recipe Color Code: | Red

Ingredients:

6 - 8 to 10 ounce fish filets of choice
1 - Tablespoon Old Bay seasoning
2 - Teaspoons paprika
1/8 - Teaspoon red pepper
1/4 - Cup plus 2 tablespoons butter or margarine, melted
1/3 - Cup lemon juice
1 - Teaspoon dried parsley flakes

Instructions:

Pre-heat broiler. Place fish filets in two lightly greased (may use non-stick cooking spray) 13" x 9" x 2" deep baking dishes, skin side down. Sprinkle Old Bay seasoning, paprika, and red pepper evenly over the fish. Brush fish with butter, sprinkle with lemon juice, and top with the parsley. Broil 109 to 12 minutes, or until fish flakes easily when tested with a fork.
Serves 4 to 6

Note: Appearance and taste are very similar to the famous blackened redfish, but much easier to prepare.

Category of Recipe: Seafood

Name of Recipe: Broiled Garlic Shrimp

Recipe Color Code: Red

Ingredients:

1 - Pound extra large shrimp (about 20) peeled and
    de-veined
2 - Tablespoons canola oil or olive oil
2 - Tablespoons dry white wine
2 - Cloves garlic, minced
2 - Medium tomatoes, halved crosswise
1/2 - Teaspoon salt
1/4 - Teaspoon ground black pepper

Instructions:

Place shrimp in a plastic bag set in a deep bowl.
Prepare marinade in a small bowl by combining the oil,
wine, garlic, salt, and pepper. Pour over the shrimp in
the bag. Close the bag. Marinate shrimp in the
refrigerator for 2 to 8 hours. Drain shrimp, reserving the
marinade. Arrange shrimp on the unheated rack of a
broiler pan. Place tomatoes, cut side up, next to shrimp.
Brush shrimp and tomatoes with marinade. Broil 4 to 6
inches from heat about 5 minutes or until shrimp turn
pink, turning shrimp over one time while cooking.
Serves 4

Category of Recipe: | Soup

Name of Recipe: | Shrimp Bisque

Recipe Color Code: | Red

Ingredients:

1 – pound shrimp, cleaned, de-veined, cooked, and chopped
½ - cup chicken broth
1 ½ - cups heavy cream
¼ - teaspoon paprika
½ - teaspoon salt
¼ - teaspoon ground black pepper
½ - cup dry sherry
1 – tablespoon parsley, chopped
1 – tablespoon chives, chopped

Instructions:

Blend ½ the shrimp and all the chicken broth in a food processor until smooth. Pour the processed mixture into the top of a double boiler. Add cream, salt, pepper, and paprika. Cook over the hot water, stirring occasionally, until the mixture almost comes to a boil. Add the remaining chopped shrimp and sherry. Serve immediately in individual cups garnished with the chives and parsley.
Serves 4 to 6

Category of Recipe:	Soup
Name of Recipe:	New England Shrimp Soup
Recipe Color Code:	Red

Ingredients:

2 - Tablespoons butter
1 - Pound shrimp; cooked, peeled and deveined
1 - Medium onion, chopped
2 - Ribs celery, chopped into bite size pieces
2 - Teaspoons dried thyme
1 - Red bell pepper, chopped
2 - Cups heavy cream
1 - Cup half and half
1/4 - Cup sherry wine
1/2 - Teaspoon salt
1/4 - Teaspoon cayenne pepper
1/4 - Teaspoon nutmeg

Instructions:

Melt 1 tablespoon butter in a skillet. Add shrimp and cook for approximately three minutes until shrimp turn pink and are done, stirring frequently to prevent scorching. Remove shrimp and set aside. In the same skillet, melt the other 1 tablespoon butter over medium heat. Add onion, celery, and thyme. Cook until vegetables are tender (about 10 minutes). Add bell pepper and cook until crisp-tender (about 5 minutes). Add remaining ingredients and 1 cup of water. Bring to boil. Add cooked shrimp and heat thoroughly but not long enough to further cook shrimp or they will be tough. Serves 4 to 6

Category of Recipe: Soup

Name of Recipe: Roasted Tomato Basil Soup

Recipe Color Code: Yellow

Ingredients:

3 – pounds ripe plum tomatoes, cut in half
¼ - cup plus 2 tablespoons virgin olive oil
1 – tablespoon kosher salt
1 ½ - teaspoons freshly ground black pepper
2 – cups yellow onions, chopped (about 2 medium)
6 – cloves garlic, minced
2 – tablespoons butter
1/4 – teaspoon crushed red pepper flakes (optional)
1 – 28 ounce can plum tomatoes, un-drained
2 – packed cups fresh basil leaves
1 – teaspoon fresh thyme leaves
1 – quart water (or chicken stock if preferred)

Instructions:

Preheat oven to 400 degrees. Toss together tomatoes, ¼ cup olive oil, salt, and pepper. Spread the tomatoes in a 1 inch layer on a baking sheet and roast 45 minutes.

In an 8-quart stockpot over medium heat, sauté the onions and garlic with 2 tablespoons olive oil, the butter, and pepper flakes for 10 minutes or until onions start to brown. Add the canned tomatoes, basil, thyme, and water. Add the oven-roasted tomatoes, including the liquid on the baking sheet. Bring to boil and simmer uncovered for 40 minutes. Pass the mixture through a food mill fitted with the coarsest blade. Taste for seasonings. Serve hot or cold.
Serves 6 to 8

Category of Recipe: | Soup

Name of Recipe: | Texas Style Beef Soup

Recipe Color Code: | Red

Ingredients:

2 - Tablespoons canola oil
3/4 - Pound beef round steak, cut into bite size cubes
1 - Large onion, chopped (approximately 1 cup)
1 - Clove garlic, minced
1 - 16 ounce can diced tomatoes, undrained
1 - 8 ounce can red kidney beans; drained and rinsed
1 - Medium green bell pepper, chopped (about 1/2 cup)
2 - Tablespoons tomato paste
1 - Tablespoon chili powder
2 - Cups beef broth
1/4 - Teaspoon ground black pepper

Instructions:

Preheat canola oil in a large sauce pan over medium
heat. Add the beef, onion, green pepper, and garlic.
Cook until beef is done as desired, stirring often to
prevent burning. Add beef broth, tomatoes, beans,
tomato paste, black pepper and chili powder. Cover and
simmer for about 30 minutes or until beef is tender.
Serves 4 to 6

Category of Recipe: Soup

Name of Recipe: Southwestern Chili

Recipe Color Code: Red

Ingredients:

2 - Medium green bell peppers, chopped
2 - Large onions, chopped
3 - Cloves garlic, minced
1 - Jalapeno pepper, finely chopped (optional)
4 - Tablespoons olive oil
1 3/4 - Pound ground beef (chuck preferred)
1 - 40 ounce can red kidney beans, drained and rinsed
1 1/2 - Teaspoons cumin
3 1/2 - Tablespoons chili powder (hot optional)
2 - Teaspoons salt
2 - 28 ounce cans diced tomatoes, undrained
1 - 28 ounce can crushed tomatoes with added puree
1 1/2 - Cup tomato juice
1 - Tablespoon Hershey's cocoa powder
4 - Packages artificial sweetener of choice
Shredded cheddar cheese for topping (optional)

Instructions:

Sauté onion, garlic, and green bell peppers in the olive oil on medium-low heat until tender, but not brown; set aside.

Place beef in a large stew pot and cook on medium-low until done; stir often to prevent burning. Drain after cooking if not low-fat beef. Add cumin, chili powder, salt, and onion mixture to beef and stir. Add tomatoes, beans jalapeno sauce, and tomato juice; stir. Add cocoa powder and sweetener; stir. Bring to slow boil; stir often. Reduce heat to low and simmer for approximately 1 hour, stirring often to prevent scorching. Serve in bowl and top with cheese.
Serves 10 to 12

Notes: This recipe makes a fantastic chili. The cocoa powder gives it a great depth of flavor and a deep chili color second to none. Hot pepper sauce may be added to a serving for those who like it hot. Try it; you will say that it deserved the ribbon that it won.

Category of Recipe: | Soup

Name of Recipe: | Cream of Mushroom Soup

Recipe Color Code: | Yellow

Ingredients:

1 - Pound fresh white mushrooms
1 - Ounce dried Morel mushrooms
3 - Tablespoons virgin olive oil
2 - Shallots, chopped
1 - Clove garlic, minced
1 - Quart hot beef broth
1/2 - Teaspoon dried thyme
Salt and pepper to taste
1/2 - Cup half and half
Fresh parsley, chopped (for garnish)

Instructions:

Soak dried Morel mushrooms in about 1 cup water for 20 minutes, then drain and reserve liquid to add extra flavor to soup. Chop the fresh white mushrooms and the Morel mushrooms. Heat the oil in a large pan and add the shallots and garlic. Cook until softened, about 5 minutes. Add both types of mushrooms and stir over moderate heat for about 5 minutes. Add the beef broth and Morel soaking liquid and bring to a boil, stirring. Add the thyme, salt and pepper. Cover and simmer for 30 minutes. In a food processor, blend about 3/4 of the mixture until smooth. Pour back into pan; add cream and season to taste. Reheat, garnish with parsley and serve immediately.
Serves 4

Category of Recipe: Soup

Name of Recipe: Southern Style Black Bean Soup

Recipe Color Code: Green

Ingredients:

1 - 1 pound package dried black beans, rinsed
6 - Cups cold tap water
1 - Tablespoon olive oil
1 - Cup celery, chopped
1 - Large onion, chopped
2 - Garlic cloves, minced
3/4 - Teaspoon dried oregano, crumbled
1 - 13 3/4 ounce can chicken broth
3 - 1/2 inch strips orange peel (do not include white part)
1 1/4 - Teaspoons salt
1/2 - Teaspoon hot pepper sauce of choice (optional)

Instructions:

In a large bowl, soak the beans overnight in 5 cups water. In a large soup pot, heat the oil over medium heat. Stir in the celery, onion, garlic and oregano; cook for 5 to 7 minutes or until the vegetables are tender. Add the soaked beans and bean liquid and the remaining 1 cup of water. Bring the mixture to a boil, reduce the heat, cover and simmer for 1 hour, stirring occasionally. Add the chicken broth, orange peel, salt, and hot pepper sauce. Cover and continue cooking for 2 or 3 hours until the beans are tender. Stir every 20 to 30 minutes to prevent the beans from sticking to the bottom of the pan. Add additional water as necessary. Makes about 9 cups. Serves 6 to 8

Category of Recipe: | Soup

Name of Recipe: | Cuban Style Black Bean Soup

Recipe Color Code: | Green

Ingredients:

1 - Pound dried black beans (2 cups)
6 - Cups water
3 - Tablespoons canola oil
1 - Large onion, finely chopped (about 1 cup)
2 - Cloves garlic, minced
1 - Stalk celery, finely chopped
1 - Teaspoon dried oregano, crumbled
1 1/2 - Teaspoons salt
1/2 - Teaspoon finely ground black pepper
1/4 - Teaspoon cayenne pepper (optional)
1/4 - Cup lemon juice
1/3 - Cup onion, chopped (for topping)

Instructions:

Remove any small rocks or unwanted beans and place others in a large bowl or crock pot. Cover with cold tap water to a depth of approximately 3 inches above the beans and soak overnight. Drain beans and place in a kettle with 6 cups fresh water. Bring to boil, cover, and simmer 2 hours, or until tender. Meanwhile, heat the oil in a medium size skillet and sauté the cup of onion until tender but not brown. Add the garlic and celery and cook 3 additional minutes. Add the oregano, salt, pepper, and cayenne. Remove 2 cups of the bean mixture and puree in an electric blender or food processor. Return to the bulk of the soup along with sautéed vegetable mixture. Reheat and taste for seasoning. Add more seasoning as desired. Add lemon juice. This should be a heavy thick mixture. Serve topped with the remaining uncooked chopped onion.
Serves 4 to 6

Category of Recipe: Soup

Name of Recipe: Cincinnati Chili

Recipe Color Code: Red

Ingredients:

1 - Tablespoon canola oil
2 - Large onions, coarsely chopped
3 - Garlic cloves, crushed
1/4 - Cup chili powder
2 - Teaspoons ground cumin
1/2 - Teaspoon salt
1/2 - Teaspoon ground cinnamon
1/4 - Teaspoon allspice
2 - Pounds lean ground beef
1 - Cup beef broth
1 - 15 ounce can tomato sauce
2 - Tablespoons tomato paste

Instructions:

In a 5 to 6 quart Dutch oven, heat oil over medium heat until hot. Add onions and cook 15 minutes or until tender; stir occasionally. Add garlic and cook 1 minute, stirring. Add chili powder, cumin, salt, cinnamon, and allspice, and cook 1 minute, stirring. Increase heat to medium-high; add ground beef and cook 12 to 15 minutes, until beef is browned and all juices have evaporated, stirring often to break up meat. Increase heat to high; add broth, tomato sauce, and tomato paste, and heat to boiling. Reduce heat to low, cover, and simmer 15 minutes to blend flavors.
Serves 8 to 10

Category of Recipe: Soup

Name of Recipe: Broccoli and Cheese Soup

Recipe Color Code: Red

Ingredients:

2 - 10 ounce packages frozen chopped broccoli
10 - Large fresh mushrooms, sliced
3 1/2 - Cups chicken broth
2 - Stalks celery, finely chopped
1/2 - Cup green onions, chopped
1 - Tablespoon fresh parsley, finely chopped
2 - Teaspoons garlic salt

Instructions:

Cook broccoli, drain and puree with 1 1/2 cups chicken broth. In a sauce pan, simmer broccoli with remaining chicken broth or stock. In a skillet, sauté vegetables in butter or margarine until tender. Season with garlic salt, add to broccoli, cover and cook for 30 minutes. Fold in cheese and sour cream. Season to taste with Worcestershire sauce. Serve immediately.
Serves 6

Category of Recipe: Soup

Name of Recipe: Virginia Beef Stew

Recipe Color Code: Red

Ingredients:

2 - Pounds beef shoulder round, cut into bite size pieces
1/3 - Cup butter
1 - Large onion, cut into wedges
1 - Cup fresh mushrooms, sliced
2 - Celery stalks, chopped
1 - Garlic clove, minced
1/4 - Teaspoon ground black pepper
1/2 - Teaspoon salt
1/2 - Cup dry red wine
2 - 10 1/2 ounce cans beef broth

Instructions:

Over medium heat, melt butter in a large deep skillet which has a lid. Add the bite size pieces of beef to the melted butter and brown. Stir frequently to prevent scorching. Add the onion, celery, mushrooms, garlic, salt and pepper. Reduce heat to medium-low and let the mixture simmer for about 25 minutes. Add the wine and beef broth. Mix, cover, and simmer for about 1hour or until the beef is done and tender.
Serves 4

Category of Recipe: Soup

Name of Recipe: Vegetable Beef Soup

Recipe Color Code: Red

Ingredients:

1 1/2 - Pounds ground chuck
3/4 - Medium head cabbage
2 - Medium onions, chopped
2 - Green bell peppers, chopped
2 - 28 ounce cans diced tomatoes
1 - 28 ounce can crushed tomatoes
2 - 15 ounce cans kidney beans, drained and rinsed
1/2 - Cup tomato juice
2 1/2 - Tablespoons chili powder
1 - Tablespoon salt
1 - Teaspoon cumin
1 - Teaspoon oregano
1 - Teaspoon hot sauce of choice (optional)

Instructions:

Chop cabbage, onions, and peppers into bit size pieces. Place in steamer and steam cook until tender. Place ground beef in a large stew pot and cook until about 75% done. Add seasonings and continue cooking until beef is completely done. Add steamed vegetables, tomato items, and kidney beans to seasoned and cooked beef. Stir. Turn stove to low heat and let simmer about 1 hour; stirring soup every 15 minutes to prevent scorching. Serves 10 to 12

Note: This has been a very popular recipe that has been refined down through the years. It is easy to prepare and absolutely delicious. I assure you that your entire family can enjoy this soup and never suspect that it is a weight loss recipe.

Category of Recipe: Soup

Name of Recipe: French Onion Soup

Recipe Color Code: Yellow

Ingredients:

3 - Cups onions, thinly sliced
1 - Tablespoon butter or margarine
2 - Packets instant beef broth mix
1 - Teaspoon Worcestershire sauce
1/8 - Teaspoon ground black pepper
2 1/2 - Ounces shredded Swiss cheese
2 1/2 - Cups water

Instructions:

In a large saucepan, combine onions and margarine; cover and cook over medium-low heat for 20 minutes, stirring occasionally. Add remaining ingredients, except cheese, and bring to a boil. Reduce heat, cover, and simmer 15 minutes. Pre-heat broiler. To serve, ladle evenly into 3 ovenproof bowls and sprinkle 1/3 of the cheese over each dish. Place under broiler until cheese is melted (about 2 minutes).
Serves 3

Category of Recipe: Soup

Name of Recipe: Gazpacho Soup

Recipe Color Code: Yellow

Ingredients:

2 - Cups cold beef broth
2 - Medium cucumbers, peeled, seeded, and finely chopped
8 - Small whole scallions, finely chopped
1 - Medium green bell pepper, finely chopped
2 - Tomatoes, finely chopped
2 - Garlic cloves, minced
1 - Cup tomato sauce
1/2 - Cup water
1 - Tablespoon red wine vinegar
1/2 - Teaspoon hot sauce of choice
2 - Teaspoons Worcester sauce
1 - Teaspoon fresh parsley, finely chopped
Salt and pepper to taste

Instructions:

Pour the beef broth into a large bowl, and then add the cumbers, scallions, green pepper, tomatoes, garlic, and tomato sauce. Water, red wine vinegar, and hot sauce. Stir until the ingredients are well combined and season with salt and pepper to taste. Chill in the refrigerator for at least 4 hours, and then add the Worcestershire sauce and parsley. Serve the gazpacho in chilled bowls.
Serves 3 to 4

Category of Recipe:	Soup

Name of Recipe:	Spanish Stew

Recipe Color Code:	Red

Ingredients:

1 - Pound smoked sausage, cut into 1/2 inch round slices
4 - Boneless and skinless chicken breast halves
1 - Pound large shrimp
2 - Tablespoons olive oil
3 - Medium onions, chopped
3 - Green bell peppers, coarsely chopped
2 - Yellow bell peppers, coarsely chopped
4 - Cloves garlic, finely chopped
1 - Tablespoon dried oregano
1 - Tablespoon dried thyme
1 - Tablespoon paprika
1 - Teaspoon salt and ½ teaspoon black pepper mixed
1 - 28 ounce can diced and peeled tomatoes with juice
1 - 14 ounce can chicken broth
1 - Cup dry white wine
4 - Packages artificial sweetener

Instructions:

Cook sausage in heavy large pot over medium heat until done. Transfer to a large bowl. Salt and pepper both sides of the chicken breasts. In olive oil, cook chicken on medium-low heat until done; turning twice. Remove chicken after cooked and cut into bite size pieces. Put in bowl with cooked sausage. Steam shrimp for 4 1/2 minutes. Immediately place cooked shrimp in colander and rinse with cold tap water to stop cooking. Peel and de-vein shrimp. Place shrimp in bowl with other meats. Cook peppers, onions, and garlic in juices of cooked chicken until tender. Stir often to avoid burning. Add oregano, thyme, and paprika; stir and sauté for about 5 more minutes. Return all three meats along with any accumulated juices, to the pot with the cooked pepper and onions. Add tomatoes, chicken broth, and wine. Stir, bring to boil, and reduce heat to a simmer. Add olives and sweetener. Stir and simmer for about 15 minutes, or until liquid is reduced to thin sauce consistency. Season to taste with salt, pepper, and hot sauce.
Serves 8 to 10

Category of Recipe: Soup

Name of Recipe: 15 Bean Soup

Recipe Color Code: Green

Ingredients:

1 - 20 ounce bag of 15 bean soup (or other dried beans)
1 - Ham hock (or other cooked meat of choice)
1 - 14 1/2 ounce can chicken broth
1 - 14 1/2 ounce can beef broth
1 - 10 ounce can RO-TEL tomatoes
1 - Cup dry white wine
1 - Teaspoon Cajun seasoning of choice (optional)
1/2 - Teaspoon ground black pepper
1 - Whole bay leaf
3 - Cups water (approximately)

Instructions:

Cover beans with approximately 3 inches of water and soak overnight. After soaking, drain and rinse beans. Place beans in crock pot. Add remaining ingredients, including the 3 cups of water. Stir well to mix. Cook in crock pot on high heat for 8 hours, or until beans are tender and the soup begins to thicken. Stir every 2 hours during the cooking time.
Serves 6 to 8

Category of Recipe: Soup

Name of Recipe: Great Gumbo

Recipe Color Code: Red

Ingredients:

1 - Pound boneless and skinless chicken breast halves
3 - Tablespoons canola oil
1/2 - Pound cooked smoked sausage, bite size pieces
2 - Medium onions, chopped
2 - Medium green bell peppers, chopped
1 - Cup celery, chopped
2 - Cups cut okra
2 - Cloves garlic, minced
1 - 28 ounce can diced tomatoes, undrained
1 - 8 ounce can tomato sauce
1 - 10 ounce can RO-TEL tomatoes with green chilies
2 - Teaspoons Worcestershire sauce
1/2 - Teaspoon dried oregano
1/2 - Teaspoon dried thyme
1 1/2 - Teaspoon salt
1 - Teaspoon Cajun seasoning of choice

Instructions:

In a large deep skillet which has a lid, heat canola oil over medium-low heat and fry the chicken until tender. Remove cooked chicken and cut into bite size pieces. Using the canola oil and juices from cooking the chicken, sauté the onion, pepper, celery, okra, and garlic until tender. Stir in tomatoes, tomato sauce, RO-TEL tomatoes, Worcestershire sauce, oregano, thyme, salt, and Cajun. Cook over medium-low heat, stirring occasionally, about 30 minutes or until desired consistency. Stir in cooked sausage, cooked chicken, and simmer over medium heat until chicken and sausage are thoroughly re-heated. Add sweetener, stir, turn heat to low and simmer for at least 30 minutes. Add hot sauce if and as desired. Stir frequently to prevent burning. Serve over cooked converted rice.
Note: To cook converted rice: To 3/4 cup water, add 1 - 14 1/2 ounce can of chicken or beef broth. Bring to boil, add 1 cup converted rice, bring back to boil and turn heat down to medium-low. Cover and cook 1 hour. DO NOT remove lid for stir while cooking or rice will stick together.
Serves 10 to 12

Category of Recipe: | Soup

Name of Recipe: | Lentil Soup

Recipe Color Code: | Green

Ingredients:

2 - Cups dried lintels, uncooked
1 - Tablespoon canola oil
1 - Cup onion, chopped
2 - Cloves garlic, minced
1 1/2 - Teaspoons curry powder
2 - 14 1/2 ounce cans beef broth (4 cups)
2 1/2 - Cups cold tap water
2 - Cups peeled and diced tomatoes
1 - Cup fresh parsley, chopped
1 - Cup permitted cooked vegetables of choice (optional)
1/2 - Cup dry red wine (optional); water or chicken stock
        if wine is omitted
Salt and pepper to taste

Instructions:

In a large sauce pan, heat oil on medium heat. Sauté onion and garlic until clear. Add curry powder and sauté for approximately 1 additional minute. Add broth, water, lentils, tomatoes, optional permitted vegetable, and the 1/2 cup of wine or water. Cover and simmer until lentils are cooked; approximately 45 minutes. Add parsley. Stir and simmer for about 5 additional minutes.
Serves 8 to 10

Note: Note: Ideal as half of a soup and salad meal.

Category of Recipe: | Soup

Name of Recipe: | Cream of Broccoli Soup

Recipe Color Code: | Red

Ingredients:

2 - 10 ounce frozen chopped broccoli, thawed and drained
1 - 14 1/2 ounce can (about 2 cups) chicken broth
1 - Small (about 1/2 cup) onion, chopped
1/2 - Cup (1 stick) margarine or butter
3/4 - Teaspoon dried basil
1 - Teaspoon salt
1/4 - Teaspoon ground black pepper
1/8 - Teaspoon ground nutmeg
1 - Tablespoon lemon juice
1 - Cup half and half cream
1/2 - Cup shredded cheddar cheese (optional for topping)

Instructions:

Remove broccoli from container, thaw, and drain (may be rapidly thawed by placing in microwaveable dish and microwaving on high for about 8 minutes). Sauté onion in butter or margarine for 5 minutes. Add broccoli, chicken broth, basil, salt, nutmeg, and pepper. Bring to simmer, cover and simmer for 15 minutes. Let cool. In a food processor, puree until smooth. Reheat mixture and add lemon juice and cream. Top with shredded cheese and serve immediately.
Serves 3 to 4

Category of Recipe:	Spreads and Dips
Name of Recipe:	Guacamole
Recipe Color Code:	Yellow

Ingredients:

4 - Ripe avocados
2 - Plum tomatoes, peeled, seeded and chopped
1 - Tablespoon onions, finely chopped
4 - Chili peppers, chopped
1 - Ounce fresh lemon juice
1 - Tablespoon Worcestershire sauce
1 - Teaspoon garlic, chopped
1 - Teaspoon salt
1/4 - Teaspoon cayenne pepper
1/2 - Teaspoon hot sauce of choice

Instructions:

Mash avocados. Coarsely chop tomatoes and chili peppers in food processor. Add avocados and al other ingredients to processor and blend until smooth. Refrigerate in covered container. Put the avocado seed in container to prevent darkening of guacamole.
Serves 8 to 10

Category of Recipe: | Spreads and Dips

Name of Recipe: | Sausage Dip

Recipe Color Code: | Red

Ingredients:

1 - 1 pound roll of sausage hot, medium, or mild to taste)
2 - 8 ounce packages cream cheese
1 - 10 ounce can RO-TEL tomatoes

Instructions:

Slice sausage into approximately 3/8 inch patties. Place patties in a large skillet and fry on medium heat until done. Remove patties and place in a plate to cool. Place the 2 packages of cream cheese in a double-boiler and heat on medium until cheese is soft and creamy (cheese may be softened in microwave). Add RO-TEL tomatoes to cheese and stir well. Place cooled sausage patties in a food processor and process until broken into small chunks (sausage may also be broken up by hand or with a fork). Add the chunks of sausage to the tomato and cheese mixture. Mix well. Serve hot. This is a good dip to be served in a mini-crock pot.
Serves 10 to 12

Category of Recipe: | Spreads and Dips

Name of Recipe: | Tomato Dip

Recipe Color Code: | Red

Ingredients:

1 - 12 ounce cream cheese, room temperature
1/4 - Cup canola oil mayonnaise
1 - Ripe tomato, quartered
1 - Celery stalk, cut into bite size pieces
2 - Garlic cloves, minced
2 - Tablespoons onion, chopped
2 - Tablespoons lemon juice
2 - Packages artificial sweetener of choice
1/2 - Teaspoon salt
1 - Teaspoon hot sauce of choice

Instructions:

Combine all ingredients in a food processor and blend until smooth. Place the dip in a serving bowl, cover and refrigerate for 2 hours. Serve with celery, green peppers, asparagus and broccoli.
Serves 8 to 10

Category of Recipe: | Spreads and Dip

Name of Recipe: | Smoked Salmon Dip or Spread

Recipe Color Code: | Red

Ingredients:

4 - Tablespoons canola oil mayonnaise
3 - Teaspoons lemon juice
2 - Teaspoons Dijon mustard
1/4 - Teaspoon salt
1 - Package artificial sweetener
1/4 - Teaspoon ground black pepper
1 1/2 - Teaspoon liquid smoke
1/2 - Teaspoon garlic, minced
1 - Teaspoon prepared horseradish
1 - 15 1/2 ounce can selected pink salmon, well drained

Instructions:

Place all ingredients in food processor and blend until smooth.
Serves 8 to 10

Note: This is an old recipe that Donald created many years ago. It has become very popular at a lot of parties.

Category of Recipe: | Vegetables

Name of Recipe: | Roasted Vegetables

Recipe Color Code: | Yellow

Ingredients:

3 – medium summer yellow squash, sliced ¼" thick
1 – pound fresh asparagus, trimmed and halved
1 – large green bell pepper, julienned
1 – large sweet red pepper, julienned
1 – medium red onion, sliced and separated into rings
5 – cups fresh cauliflowerets
5 – cups fresh broccoli florets
¼ - cup virgin olive oil
3 – tablespoons lemon juice
2 – garlic cloves, minced
1 – tablespoon dried rosemary, crushed
1 – teaspoon salt
½ - teaspoon ground black pepper

Instructions:

Preheat oven to 400 degrees. In a large bowl, combine all vegetables. In a small bowl, whisk the oil, lemon juice, garlic, rosemary, salt, and pepper until well blended. Drizzle mixture over vegetables and toss to coat. Transfer to two greased 15 inch by 10 inch baking pans. Bake, uncovered, at 400 degrees for 20 to 25 minutes or until vegetables are tender, occasionally stirring.
Serves 10 to 12

You will be very pleased by the many compliments from your guests when you serve these delicious veggies.

Category of Recipe:	Vegetables
Name of Recipe:	Broccoli with Cheese Sauce
Recipe Color Code:	Red

Ingredients:

1 1/2 - Pounds fresh broccoli
1/2 - Teaspoon dried oregano
1/2 - Teaspoon salt
1/2 - Cup sugar-free mayonnaise
1/3 - Cup shredded cheddar cheese
1/4 - Cup low fat milk
2 - Tablespoons grated Parmesan cheese

Instructions:

Trim off large leaves of broccoli and remove tough ends; wash thoroughly and cut into spears. Place broccoli in a shallow 2 quart baking dish, with stem ends toward outside the dish; sprinkle oregano on top and add 1/2 cup water. Cover with lid or heavy duty vented plastic wrap and microwave on high power for 8 minutes. Stir and cook an additional 3 minutes on high power or until tender. Drain and place in a serving dish. Sprinkle with salt, if desired. Combine the mayonnaise, cheddar cheese, and milk in a 1 or 2 cup glass measuring cup. Microwave on medium power (70%) for 1 minute; stir, and cook an additional minute or until cheese melts. Stir again a spoon mixture over broccoli. Sprinkle with Parmesan cheese over sauce.
Serves 4

Category of Recipe: | Vegetables

Name of Recipe: | Cajun Vegetable Jambalaya

Recipe Color Code: | Yellow

Ingredients:

1/2 - Cup canola oil
3 - Medium onions, chopped
2 - Tablespoons shallots, chopped
2 - Medium green bell peppers, chopped
1 - Large eggplant, peeled and chopped (about 2 cups)
3 - Yellow squash, chopped (about 2 cups)
2 - Cloves garlic, minced
4 - Tomatoes, chopped (about 3 cups)
3 - Teaspoons salt
1 - Teaspoons cayenne pepper
2 - Teaspoons hot sauce of choice
3 - Bay leaves
3 - Cups converted rice
6 - Cups water
1 - Cup green onions, chopped

Instructions:

Heat the oil in a large heavy pot over medium heat. Add the onions, shallots, bell peppers, eggplant, squash and garlic. Sauté until tender, about 4 minutes. Add the tomatoes. Season with salt, cayenne, and hot sauce. Add the bay leaves. Add the rice and stir for 3 minutes. Add the water, stir and cover. Cook for 35 minutes or until the rice is tender and the liquid has been absorbed. Do not stir during this cooking time. Remove from heat and let stand for 3 minutes. Add the green onions and mix.
Serves 8 to 10

Category of Recipe: Vegetables

Name of Recipe: Asparagus with Buttered Hazelnuts

Recipe Color Code: Yellow

Ingredients:

1/2 - Tablespoon butter, plus
1 - Tablespoon butter
2 - Tablespoon hazelnuts, chopped
1 - Pound asparagus, trimmed
1 - Teaspoon dried thyme
1 - Teaspoon fresh parsley, chopped
1 - Teaspoon lemon juice
1/2 - Teaspoon salt
1/4 - Teaspoon ground black pepper

Instructions:

In a large skillet, melt 1/2 tablespoon butter over medium heat. Add hazelnuts and cook until toasted; remove. In same skillet, over medium heat, melt remaining butter. Add asparagus and cook until just crisp-tender, about 5 minutes. Add remaining ingredients, sprinkle with buttered hazelnuts and serve.
Serves 4

Category of Recipe: | Vegetables

Name of Recipe: | Marinated Vegetables

Recipe Color Code: | Yellow

Ingredients:

3/4 - Cup olive oil
3/4 - Cup canola oil
1 - Teaspoon salt
2 - Teaspoons dry mustard
4 - Packages artificial sweetener
1/2 - Cup red wine vinegar
1 - Small onion, chopped
3 - Ribs celery, cut into bite size pieces
2 - Green bell pepper, cut into bite size pieces
4 - Ounces mushrooms, sliced
1 - Bunch cauliflower, cut into bite size pieces
1 - Bunch broccoli, cut into florets

Instructions:

Blanch broccoli and cauliflower in a large pot of boiling water until just barely tender. Drain and rise with cold water. In a large bowl, combine broccoli, cauliflower, mushrooms, pepper, celery and onion. In a medium bowl, combine the vinegar, sweetener, mustard, salt and vegetable oil. Mix until well blended. Pour the marinade over the vegetables and mix well. Chill overnight before serving. Keep any extras refrigerated.
Serves 10 to 12

Category of Recipe: | Vegetables

Name of Recipe: | Cabbage Lasagna

Recipe Color Code: | Red

Ingredients:

1 - Medium head cabbage, cut into large chunks
1 - Medium onion, chopped
1 - Green pepper, chopped
1 - 6 ounce can V-8 juice
1 - Teaspoon dry Italian seasoning
1/2 - Teaspoon garlic powder
1 - Pound ground lean beef
1 - Cup shredded Mozzarella cheese

Instructions:

Pre-heat oven to 350 degrees. In a steamer, or by boiling, cook cabbage until tender. In a saucepan, combine onion, green pepper, V-8 juice, Italian seasoning, and garlic powder. Bring to boil and lower heat to simmer while cooking ground beef. In a large skillet, cook ground beef and drain off liquids. Add cooked ground beef to sauce; stir well. Spray a 9" x 13" baking dish with a non-stick spray. Place cooked cabbage in bottom of baking dish; distribute evenly. Top cooked cabbage with the prepared meat sauce. Sprinkle Mozzarella cheese over top of meat sauce. Bake at 350 degrees for 30 minutes.
Serves 8

Note: This recipe is a great meal by itself!

Category of Recipe: | Vegetables

Name of Recipe: | Quick-top Cauliflower

Recipe Color Code: | Yellow

Ingredients:

1 - Small head cauliflower (approximately 1 pound)
3 - Tablespoons Italian dressing
2 1/4 - Ounces shredded cheddar cheese
1/4 - Cup sugar-free mayonnaise
2 - Tablespoons onion, finely chopped
1 - Teaspoon prepared mustard
1/4 - Cup water
Fresh parsley, chopped for garnish (optional)

Instructions:

In a 2 1/2 quart microwavable casserole dish, place the head of cauliflower and 1/4 cup water. Sprinkle with the Italian dressing. Cover tightly with vented plastic wrap. Microwave on high power for 9 minutes, or until cauliflower is tender. In a small bowl, combine cheese, mayonnaise, onion, and mustard; spread mixture evenly over cauliflower. Microwave, uncovered, and on high power for 3 minutes, or until cheese is melted. Let stand for 1 minute, garnish with parsley if desired.
Serves 4

Category of Recipe: | Vegetables

Name of Recipe: | Broccoli with Cheese and Butter Sauce

Recipe Color Code: | Red

Ingredients:

1 - Tablespoon butter
1/2 - Pound broccoli florets
1/2 - Teaspoon ground black pepper, divided
1/4 - Teaspoon salt
4 - Ounces shredded cheddar cheese
1/2 - Cup heavy cream
1/2 - Teaspoon dry mustard
1/4 - Teaspoon paprika
1 - Egg yolk

Instructions:

In a skillet, melt butter over medium heat. Add broccoli and cook until crisp-tender; 6 to 8 minutes. Season with 1/4 teaspoon pepper and salt. To prepare cheese sauce: In pot combine cheese, cream, mustard, paprika, remaining pepper and 1/4 cup water. Cook over medium-low heat until cheese melts. In a bowl, gradually whisk 2 tablespoons hot cheese mixture into egg yolk. Gradually whisk yolk-cheese mixture into cheese mixture; cook until cheese sauce thickens. Drizzle broccoli with cheese sauce and serve.
Serves 8

Category of Recipe: | Vegetables

Name of Recipe: | Sautéed Vegetable Combo

Recipe Color Code: | Yellow

Ingredients:

2 - Tablespoons canola oil
1 - Medium onion, thinly sliced
1 - Medium green bell pepper, thinly sliced
1 - Clove garlic, minced
2 - Medium zucchini squash, thinly sliced
2 - Medium yellow summer squash, thinly sliced
3 - Cups fresh spinach leaves
1/4 - Teaspoon ground cumin
1/4 - Teaspoon salt
1/8 - Teaspoon ground black pepper

Instructions:

Heal oil in a large skillet over medium-high heat. Add onion, bell pepper, and garlic. Cook and stir 2 to 3 minutes or until crisp-tender. Stir in zucchini, summer squash, spinach, cumin salt, and pepper. Cook and stir 3 to 4 additional minutes or until squash is crisp-tender and mixture is thoroughly heated.
Serves 3 to 4

Category of Recipe:	Vegetables

Name of Recipe:	Stir Fry Vegetables

Recipe Color Code:	Yellow

Ingredients:

1/4 - Cup canola oil
2 - Cups Chinese cabbage, coarsely shredded
1 - Cup green bell pepper, sliced into about 1/4 inches each
1 - 16 ounce can bean sprouts, drained
1 - 8 ounce can sliced water chestnuts, drained
1 - 8 ounce can bamboo shoots, drained
3 - Cups spinach, coarsely chopped
2 - Tablespoons soy sauce
1/2 - Teaspoon salt

Instructions:

Heat electric wok or skillet at 350 degrees for 2 to 3 minutes. Add oil and heat for 1 minute. Add shredded cabbage, sliced green pepper, bean sprouts, bamboo shoots and water chestnuts to oil in wok. Stir fry vegetables for 5 minutes. Cover wok, and cook vegetables over low heat for 3 to 5 minutes. Stir in chopped spinach, soy sauce, and salt. Stir fry vegetable mixture about 2 additional minutes or until spinach wilts. Serves 6

Category of Recipe: Vegetables

Name of Recipe: Squash Medley

Recipe Color Code: Yellow

Ingredients:

3 - Tablespoons olive oil
1 - Medium onion, thinly sliced
1 - Large zucchini, thinly sliced
4 - Medium yellow squash, thinly sliced
1 - Medium green bell pepper, cut into thin strips
1 - Teaspoon salt
1/2 - Teaspoon ground black pepper
3 - Medium tomatoes, peeled and quartered
1/2 - Cup grated Parmesan cheese

Instructions:

Place olive oil in a large skillet, coating sides and bottom.
Heat for 2 minutes on medium heat. Add onion and
green pepper, stir fry on medium heat for about 3
minutes. Add zucchini and yellow squash. Cook for an
additional 3 to 4 minutes on medium heat until tender
crisp. Add tomatoes, salt, and pepper; stir well. Remove
from heat, sprinkle cheese over vegetables, and toss
gently until cheese melts.
Serves 4 to 6

Category of Recipe: Vegetables

Name of Recipe: Squash Medley with Herbs

Recipe Color Code: Yellow

Ingredients:

3 - Medium yellow squash
3 - Medium zucchini squash
1/4 - Cup olive oil
4 - Green onions, white part only, sliced
1/4 - Teaspoon dried basil
1/4 - Teaspoon dried oregano
1/4 - Teaspoon dried thyme
1/4 - Teaspoon dried rosemary
2 - Tablespoons red wine vinegar
1 - Teaspoon salt
1/4 - Teaspoon ground black pepper
1 - Cup water

Instructions:

Thoroughly wash squash and cut into about 1/2 inch cubes. Place in a large saucepan with 1 cup water. Cover. Cook over high heat for about 6 minutes. Stir two or three times during cooking. When just tender, drain in colander and set aside. In a skillet, heat olive oil over medium heat. Stir in green onions. Sauté until transparent. Add herbs and vinegar; mix. Add the squash. Season with salt and black pepper. Toss until thoroughly mixed and heat. Serve hot or warm.
Serves 4

Category of Recipe: | Vegetables

Name of Recipe: | Buttered Yellow Squash

Recipe Color Code: | Red

Ingredients:

3 - Medium yellow squash
1/3 - Stick butter or margarine
1/4 - Medium onion, diced
Salt and pepper to taste

Instructions:

Wash squash, trim off ends, and slice into about 1/8 inch slices. Heat butter, on medium-low heat, in a deep skillet which can be covered with a lid, until butter is melted. Put diced onions into melted butter and cover the skillet with a lid. Sauté on medium-low heat for about 5 minutes, stirring twice. Place sliced squash in skillet and turn to coat with butter. Place lid on skillet and cook on medium-low heat for approximately 20 minutes or until tender, occasionally stirring for even cooking of the slices. Salt and pepper to taste.
Serves 3 to 4

Category of Recipe: | Vegetables

Name of Recipe: | Spaghetti Squash

Recipe Color Code: | Yellow

Ingredients:

1 - Medium spaghetti squash

Instructions:

Cut squash lengthwise and remove seeds. Bake cut-side down 45 minutes at 350 degrees, turn, and bake till the skin is tender (or, microwave on high power, cut-side down, for 14 minutes in 1/4 cup of water, covered with clear wrap. Using fork, release spaghetti-like strands of cooked squash. Add salt, pepper, bacon bits, butter, Parmesan cheese, etc., or, serve as pasta with spaghetti sugar-free sauce of choice.
Serves 2 to 3

Category of Recipe:	Vegetables

Name of Recipe:	Butternut Squash with Coconut Casserole

Recipe Color Code:	Red

Ingredients:

1 - Large butternut squash (about 2 cups cooked)
2 - Large eggs, beaten
1/2 - Cup milk
2 - Tablespoons plus 2 teaspoons margarine, melted
4 - Tablespoons coconut, shredded
1 - Teaspoon vanilla extract
1/2 - Teaspoon ground ginger
3 - Packages artificial sweetener
1/2 - Teaspoon ground nutmeg

Instructions:

Wash any dirt from the squash and pierce the skin several times, all around the squash, with a fork or a knife. Place 2 paper towels in the microwave with the squash on the towels. Cook squash on high power for 6 minutes. Turn the squash over and cook on high power for an additional 6 minutes. When cooked, let cool, then cut in half, lengthwise. Remove seeds with a spoon. Remove the cooked squash from the skin and place the cooked squash in a large mixing bowl and mash. Combine all the other ingredients and stir into the cooked squash until all are thoroughly blended. Spray a 9" x 5" (with deep sides) microwavable baking dish with a non-stick cooking spray and place the squash mixture in the dish. Microwave, uncovered, on medium power for 12 minutes; then on high power, cook for an additional 3 minutes until firm (or you may pre-heat the oven to 350 degrees and bake uncovered for 45 minutes). Let stand 2 minutes before serving.
Serves 2 to 4

Category of Recipe: | Vegetables

Name of Recipe: | Spinach Cheese Loaf

Recipe Color Code: | Red

Ingredients:

1 - 10 ounce package frozen chopped spinach, thawed
      and drained
16 - Ounces sharp cheddar cheese
1/2 - Cup chopped pecans, toasted (for garnish)
1/2 - Cup canola oil mayonnaise
2 - 8 ounce packages cream cheese, softened and
      divided
1/4 teaspoon salt
1/4 teaspoon ground black pepper
1/4 cup chutney
1/4 teaspoon ground nutmeg

Instructions:

Line a 9 inch by 5 inch loaf pan with heave duty plastic wrap. Press spinach between layers of paper towels to remove excess moisture; set aside. Stir together cheddar cheese, pecans, and mayonnaise. Spread half of the mixture evenly into the prepared pan. Stir together spinach, 1 package of cream cheese, salt, and pepper; spread evenly over cheddar cheese layer. Stir together remaining package of cream cheese, chutney, and nutmeg; spread evenly over spinach layer. Top with remaining cheddar cheese mixture. Cover and freeze. Will keep well for up to 1 month. Thaw in refrigerator overnight. Garnish, if desired, and serve.
Serves 6 to 8

Category of Recipe: Vegetables

Name of Recipe: Sautéed Peppers and Onions

Recipe Color Code: Yellow

Ingredients:

2 - Sweet red bell peppers, cut into 1/4 inch strips
2 - Green bell peppers, cut into 1/4 inch strips
1 - Large onion, sliced and separated into rings
1 - Clove garlic, crushed
3 - Tablespoons olive oil
1/2 - Teaspoon salt
1/2 - Teaspoon dried whole basil
1/4 - Teaspoon freshly ground black pepper

Instructions:

Sauté peppers, onion, and garlic in ho oil just until tender. Stir in salt, basil, and pepper.
Serves 4 to 6

Category of Recipe: Vegetables

Name of Recipe: Sautéed Mushrooms in Sour Cream

Recipe Color Code: Red

Ingredients:

1 - Pound fresh mushrooms, sliced
2 - Medium onions, finely chopped (about 1 cup)
1/4 - Cup margarine or butter
1 - Cup sour cream
1 - Teaspoon dill weed
1/4 - Teaspoon garlic powder
1/2 - Teaspoon salt
1/4 - Teaspoon ground black pepper

Instructions:

Melt the margarine or butter in a frying pan over medium heat. Add the onion and sauté until tender. Add the sliced mushrooms and continue to sauté until the mixture is lightly brown. Add the remaining ingredients. Stir and sauté until all the ingredients are thoroughly heated. Add salt and pepper. Stir and serve immediately.
Serves 4

Category of Recipe: | Vegetables

Name of Recipe: | Eggplant Parmigiania

Recipe Color Code: | Red

Ingredients:

1 - Medium eggplant peeled and cut into 3/8 inch slices.
Salt (for sprinkling on eggplant slices)
3 - Tablespoons olive oil (to sauté onion)
1/2 - Cup canola oil (for frying eggplant slices)
1 - Clove garlic, finely chopped
1 - Large onion, finely chopped (about 1 cup)
1 - 28 ounce can peeled and diced tomatoes, drained
1 - 14 1/2 ounce can peeled and diced tomatoes, drained
1 - Teaspoon leaf basil, crumbled
1 - Teaspoon leaf oregano, crumbled
1 - Teaspoon salt (for tomato sauce)
1/2 - Teaspoon freshly ground black pepper
1/2 - Teaspoon nutmeg
3 - Eggs, lightly beaten
1 1/2 - Cups shredded mozzarella cheese
1/2 - Cup (2 ounces) freshly grated Parmesan cheese

Instructions:

Sprinkle both sides of eggplant slices with salt and let stand 30 minutes. Meanwhile, heat 3 tablespoons olive oil in a heavy saucepan and sauté the garlic and onion until tender but not browned. Add tomatoes and cook over high heat for 15 minutes to thicken. Preheat oven to 350 degrees. Add basil, oregano, salt, pepper, and nutmeg. Cook over moderate heat for 10 minutes. Rinse off the eggplant slices and dry them on paper towels. Dip slices in the beaten egg. Heat 1/4 cup canola oil in a heavy skillet and fry the slices on both sides and in a single layer until lightly browned. Add more oil if necessary. Drain cooked slices on towels. Spray and 8" x 10" baking dish with a non-stick cooking spray, and cover the bottom with 4 tablespoons of the cooked tomato sauce and alternate layers as follows; eggplant, tomato sauce, mozzarella cheese, and Parmesan cheese (ending with the mozzarella cheese topped with Parmesan). Bake at 350 degree for 22 minutes or until bubbly hot and the top cheese has melted. Let stand 1- to 15 minutes before serving.
Serves 4 to 6

Category of Recipe: | Vegetables

Name of Recipe: | Romano Topped Tomatoes

Recipe Color Code: | Red

Ingredients:

3 - Tomatoes, halved crosswise
1 - Teaspoon salt
1/2 - Teaspoon ground black pepper
2 - Tablespoons butter or margarine
2 - Tablespoons fresh parsley, chopped
2 - Tablespoons grated Romano cheese
Fresh parsley sprigs

Instructions:

Sprinkle cut side of tomato halves with salt and pepper.
Microwave on high power, uncovered, for 3 minutes or
until thoroughly heated. Place 1 teaspoon butter, 1
teaspoon parsley, and 1 teaspoon cheese on each half.
Microwave on high power for an additional 1 1/2 minutes.
Place a tomato half on a serving plate and place a few
parsley sprigs around the tomato for appearance.
Serves 4 to 6

PERMITTED FOODS

NOTE: Refer to the previous "**GUIDE FOR USING THE RECIPE AND FOOD CHOICE COLOR CODES**" on page "17" for the descriptions of, along with detailed instructions on how to use, the below color codes.

Food Item	Color Code
Almond	Yellow
Apple juice, unsweetened	Green
Apple muffin, small	Yellow
Apple, fresh medium, no more than one	Green
Apricots, dried	Green
Apricots, fresh, medium, no more than two	Green
Artichokes	Green
Asparagus	Green
Avocado	Green
Bacon	Red
Baked Beans	Green
Barley, boiled	Yellow
Beans, Green; raw or cooked	Green
Beef, any cut	Red
Black Beans, boiled	Yellow
Black-eyed Peas, canned; recommend draining and rinsing	Yellow
Bok Choy, raw	Green

Bologna .... Red

Brazil Nuts.. Yellow

Bread, Ezekiel 4.9 made from sprouts, wheat free .... Red

Bread, pumpernickel rye .... Yellow

Broccoli, raw or cooked .... Green

Bulgur, boiled .... Yellow

Butter .... Red

Butter Beans; drain and rinse if canned .... Yellow

Cabbage, raw or cooked .... Green

Cake, sponge, plain without topping of any kind .... Yellow

Capellini pasta, boiled .... Yellow

Carrots, raw or peeled and boiled .... Yellow

Cashew Nuts .... Yellow

Cauliflower, raw or cooked .... Green

Celery .... Green

Cheese, any variety .... Red

Cherries, raw, unsweetened .... Green

Chicken noodle soup .... Yellow

Chicken Nuggets .... Red

Chickpeas; drain and rinse if canned .... Yellow

Chocolate Pudding .... Red

Coconut .... Yellow

Cottage Cheese .... Red

Crabmeat .... Red

Cucumber .... Green

Custard .... Red

Dates, Dried .... Yellow

Eggs, any style .... Red

Fettuccine .... Yellow

Fish, any species, cooked any way; including fish sticks .... Red

Garlic .... Yellow

Grapefruit juice, unsweetened .... Green

Grapefruit, raw; or canned if unsweetened .... Green

Grapes, fresh .... Green

Greens, any type .... Green

Ham .... Red

Hamburger (ground beef or turkey), without bun .... Red

Hazelnuts .... Yellow

Hot dogs; no bun .... Red

Ice Cream, artificial sweetener or no sugar added; vanilla only............... Red

Kidney Beans, fresh cooked or if canned, drained and rinsed ....Yellow

Lamb, any cut .... Red

Lemons .... Green

Lentils, fresh boiled or canned; drain and rinse if canned .... Yellow

Lettuce .... Green

Lima Beans .... Yellow

Limes .... Green

Linguine pasta .... Yellow

Lobster .... Red

Macadamia nuts .... Yellow

Macaroni with tomatoes...Yellow

Macaroni, cooked; avoid cheese or cream mixed in .... Yellow

Mango .... Green

Margarine made from 100% canola oil .... Yellow

Margarine, regular .... Red

Milk, butter .... Red

Milk, chocolate .... Red

Milk, whole, 2% or skimmed .... Red

Mousse, any flavor .... Red

Muesli, with 2% milk only .... Red

Mung Beans .... Yellow

Mustard .... Green

Navy Beans .... Yellow

Noodles, boiled; without cream, butter or cheese .... Yellow

Oatmeal; made with rolled oats only .... Yellow

Oranges, fresh; avoid orange juice .... Green

Oysters, raw or cooked .... Red

Peaches, fresh; avoid canned .... Green

Peanuts, dry roasted; avoid boiled .... Yellow

Pears, fresh; avoid canned .... Green

Peas, fresh, frozen or canned .... Green

Pecans .... Yellow

Peppers, red or green .... Green

Pickles; any style .... Green

Pineapple juice, unsweetened; avoid fresh raw pineapple .... Green

Pinto Beans, dried and boiled or canned; drain and rinse if canned .... Yellow

Plums, raw .... Green

Pork, any cut .... Red

Prunes (dried plums) .... Green

Pudding, instant; made from powder and whole milk .... Red

Rice, brown, steamed .... Yellow

Rice, Converted, white, boiled .... Yellow

Rice, long grain, boiled .... Yellow

Salami .... Red

Sausages, fried, any style .... Red

Shrimp, fried, steamed, boiled, or grilled.. Red

Soy milk .... Yellow

Soybeans, dried, fresh boiled, or canned .... Yellow

Spaghetti, whole wheat .... Yellow

Spinach, raw or cooked .... Green

Split peas, dried and boiled; avoid split pea soup .... Yellow

Squash, any type, raw or cooked .... Green

Sunflower seeds .... Yellow

Sushi .... Red

Sweet potato, baked; avoid all toppings .... Yellow

Tomato juice, no sugar added .... Green

Tomato ketchup .... Green

Tomato soup .... Green

Tomatoes .... Green

Tuna .... Red

Turkey .... Red

Veal .... Red

Vegetable soup .... Green

Walnuts .... Yellow

Wine, red or white .... Green

Yams, pealed and boiled .... Yellow

Yogurt, any flavor .... Red

Helpful Guides

WEIGHT AND MEASURE EQUIVALENTS

Dash or pinch = less than 1/8 teaspoon

3 teaspoons = 1 tablespoon or ½ fluid ounce

2 tablespoons = 1/8 cup or 1 fluid ounce

4 tablespoons = ¼ cup or 2 fluid ounces

5 tablespoons plus 1 teaspoon = 1/3 cup

8 tablespoons = ½ cup

10 2/3 tablespoons = 2/3 cup

12 tablespoons = ¾ cup

16 tablespoons = 1 cup or 8 fluid ounces or ½ pint

7/8 cup = ¾ cup plus 2 tablespoons

2 cups = 1 pint or 16 fluid ounces

4 cups = 2 pints or 1 quart or 32 fluid ounces

4 quarts = 1 gallon or 128 ounces

8 quarts = 1 peck

4 pecks = 1 bushel

16 ounces = 1 pound

SUGGESTED SIMPLE SERVING SIZE GUIDE FOR WEIGHT CONTROL

Type Food	Portion
Meat, poultry or fish	Size of the palm of your hand
Grains	A large handful
Nuts	A small handful
Vegetables	Amount equal to size of your fist
Fruits	Amount about size of a baseball
Milk	1 cup
Cheese	Size of two dominos
Wine	1 glass